THE MUSINGS OF A SCHIZO-PHRENIC TRUCK DRIVER

By
Albert M. Wessel

𝔉

Creating Forward Press

Copyright © 2021 by Albert Michel Wessel

All rights reserved. No part of this book may be reproduced in any manner whatsoever without written permission except in the case of brief quotations embodied in critical articles and reviews.

ISBN# 978-0-9869489-3-0

*"Neither a lofty degree
of intelligence
nor
imagination
nor both together
go to the making of genius.
Love, Love, Love,
that is the soul of genius."*

Wolfgang Amadeus Mozart

Once upon a time
in a mythical land
a child was born

A boy child
Beautiful of body and disposition

Loved by family
and all who knew him

But this was a terrible time of warring
and there was much fear in the land

And it came to pass
when the boy was of two years
the family
in fear for their lives
did flee their home
to a distant land
where a strange tongue was spoken

And the boy did run
from the people of the new land
and did not speak

The parents sought help for their child
but
woe of woes
were told
that their child would never speak

The years went by
and the boy grew into a young man

He never spoke
and shunned all not of family

And it came to pass
that a close friend of the family
who worked as a professional in such matters
slowly befriended the young man

And more
the friend believed in freedom
and became dedicated to the young man
And the friend did many things
to make it possible for the young man to work

And so it was
with constant support
and by the grace,
help, and encouragement of others,
the young man learned to drive a truck

He could not leave the safety of a home
so a special compartment was built
so that he could live in the truck

And it came to pass
that the young man felt safe in his new environment
and lived in contentment

The situation became well known
and all the truckers protectively watched over him
and accepted him as one of their own

Through difficulties and breakdown
there was always someone to help

The years went by

The only trauma was replacing a truck

for this was home and security

But the old friend was always there
for these huge adjustments

And the years went by

And the man listened to the radio

He learned and learned
and in this safe environment
he secretly made sounds
and began to speak to himself

He had heard others whisper
that he could not speak or read

And through his great fear
believed that he wasn't allowed
to speak or read

So he spoke
read
listened and learned
very secretly

And then he did listen to a radio station
with words only of the spiritual

He loved the biblical words

He found the radio voice to have a different
explanation
than he thought to be so

But the whispers too

had told
that there was something wrong with his head

So he believed
that everything he would think must be wrong

And the old friend did visit the man many times

And it happened one day that the man forgot
and did speak a word in front of his old friend

He hid his head
believing that he must not speak

But the old friend finally made him believe that
speaking was good

And the man spoke words to his friend

And the man so trusted his friend
that he told of his speaking in the truck
and of his childish game of pretending to be
speaking to many people

And then the man told of what he really believed
for deep down he felt that his thoughts were right

He had been forty years alone
trying to understand

And slowly the old friend helped the man to leave
the truck

And to speak to someone else

And so it was

still with great fear
the man began to speak his words
to a few people close to his old friend

And lo
a miracle
the fear was gone

And it came to pass
that the man traveled throughout the land
speaking his truths

for this was a time of great change
and the people hungered and thirsted for knowing

And the man lived happily ever after

INTRODUCTION

Encouragement to read was the greatest gift I received from my father. Where one may reap and sow, I read and sowed, all thanks to my father.

A story in the 4th-grade reader revealed this principle. It spoke of a man, his orchard, and his three sons. The sons were lazy and the father struggled to get them to work. But then the father died. Eagerly and tirelessly, the sons read their father's Last Will and Testament, which explained that there was a pot of gold buried in the orchard. The sons went right to work. They dug everywhere but could not find the gold. At first, they were just frustrated with all of their labor but they began to grow angry. They grew angry for the fruitless labor and then angrier at their father and his deception. Yet, as a result of this incidental cultivation, the orchard gave forth a rich harvest for which the sons received a pot of gold.

Such is the nature of teaching and learning and such is the nature of the spiritual harvest.

My father also taught me hard work – fence installation, tilling the garden, and automobile repair to name just a few. Installing a fence is quite a simple thing really - dig a hole in the ground, put a post in it, shovel the dirt around the post, and finally - the part that requires care, and on which my father put a great emphasis - tamp material around the post. The key is to tamp the first little bit very well. With this first hard tamping, less tamping is required for the additional layers. No amount of tamping on the higher layers will make the post secure if the first little bit isn't done well.

My father also encouraged me to explore. I climbed layers of the dry, tamped ground through sagebrush and greenery as many farm boys did in Westwold, British Columbia – mountain climbing, that is. I climbed to explore from the top. But on my first trek, to my surprise, I hadn't reached the top. From the peak of that mountain that skirted our farm, I discovered a small vale and a higher rise that had been hidden from my view. After some disappointment and contemplation, I climbed the higher mountain as well. But from that higher point, I found a small valley and a still higher mountain beyond. This realization was too much for me and I went home disappointed. But I never forgot the shock of horizons leading to horizons, leading to more horizons.

Nor have I forgotten the restrictions of a limited point of view.

I consider myself to have been born into privilege, a type of privilege that has nothing to do with financial wealth. With a firsthand understanding of the importance of a good start and seeing the danger of a limited point of view, I realized that horizons are there to lead us to further horizons. My glimpse of the road to spiritual knowledge and hidden meaning was my learning tool and I was privileged. And on top of it all, I was obsessed with reading, how could I go wrong?

There, that pretty well covers my personal history, except for the very beginning, but I'll cover that later after a little detour of about seventy years, most of which is much too boring to cover – although I pondered the meaning of ordinary things, I was partially engaged in the ordinary.

I wonder if there is something wrong with this whole learning thing. Maybe it's not just me. Maybe there is something wrong with the system. What is this business of spending a lifetime learning about life? How come we don't start with an understanding of life so that we can get right on with it? We spend a lifetime learning how life works and then what?

I can see spending a month or so learning how to drive and that's a good investment of time. But spending 70 years to understand how to operate your life is not a good ratio even if you live to 140 - especially when you consider that it's harder to dance and climb mountains in the later years.

Something doesn't add up here. I'll learn for 5 or 10 years, or even until the body gets to full size, but any more than that and you have to wonder if it's worth it or whether we might have missed something, somewhere along the way.

I will now end with the beginning: What if we could go back and look at life from the perspective of a child? Could it be that we start with everything we need to know built right into our system but we have no way to articulate that knowing because those faculties for articulation aren't yet developed? And more, could it be that in the process of developing those faculties, we conform to the world instead of learning how to articulate our innate wisdom? Do we learn to perpetuate the ways of the world rather than the wisdom we were born with?

Well then, if we answer in the affirmative to the above questions, our main concern in caring for those who are at the beginning of life must be to find ways to allow inherent knowing to flourish. That's what's missing. How can we expect to be functional without that all-important wisdom we brought with us?

We cannot and we do not function anywhere near optimum. Nor can we go back and redo our childhood so that we can restart at an optimum level. But what if we could be privy to a child's wisdom?

A newborn lives in joy, knowing nothing of the difficulties of this world. Everything is provided for. The baby has no worries and has no concept of anything but bliss. All is well and the baby mostly sleeps or gazes around in wonder and learns little things like moving parts of its body. And there are always at least two loving hands to care for every need - not to mention that warm, wonderful nourishment direct from mother's body complete with that intimate embrace that leaves no room for even a query of anything other than a wonderful world where all things are quite naturally forthcoming. The child knows only joy. It has no frame of reference for anything else. Indeed, the infant has it right. This is quite the natural order of the universe.

But that's not quite the order we have created here on earth and things do change for this infant: Time goes by and once in a while a need is not fulfilled immediately and minor discomforts are experienced. More time goes by, although time is certainly not a concept. Experiencing small discomforts increase a little, but the baby has learned that making a noise usually brings somebody to make it all right. So, everything is still fine in this child's life. But eventually, what gets the baby's attention are the sounds the big people are making. With a lot of repetition, the baby begins to understand and distinguish one sound from another.

Understanding words is a giant leap! A different kind of communication is beginning to take place. This business of using words is very exciting and the child is thrilled with the newfound ability - and so is everyone else. A new dimension has been added. Now the child starts to understand the words that accompany the feelings of love that he receives from his parents. Words enhance what is being communicated by other means. Things just keep getting better in this child's world.

As progress is made, the child learns words that are used for his protection. He understands the word no, and he feels that it is used in love to keep him from harm. He is starting to understand how our world functions. With words, the ways of the world are communicated to this new member of the world - a very necessary process.

But there comes a time, not long after learning to talk, that a child begins to disobey. This usually starts to happen around age two and can escalate to an unreasonable level. Any parent can tell you about a dear little angel turning into a holy terror around that age. It's called the terrible two's and for a very good reason.

The first do's and don'ts he is exposed to are fine, but it's just a matter of time before he comes across do's and don'ts that do not feel good to him. He is not just being contrary. The problem is that some of the no's he is coming against feel wrong to him. As much as he instinctively understands what is in his own best interest, he also instinctively understands what is *against* his true nature. Of course, he certainly can't put that knowing into words, but it is a very strong knowing that he cannot ignore. He is still operating exclusively from a knowing that doesn't have words. He does not yet think in words. But some of the communication coming to him is bothering him a lot. Some of what he is being told is in sharp opposition to that innate knowing he was born with. The implication of what he is being asked to do is unacceptable. And so he reacts.

We could get stuck at this impasse, but the real kicker for the child is the world beyond the immediate family. That's where the artificial niceties of the outer world are revealed - revealed to be in stark contrast to his inner world.

He doesn't like Aunt Ester and he freely expresses that dislike. Aunt Ester has bad breath and so the child tells her she stinks. But he is told that a good little boy doesn't say things like that. Still, he knows full well that Aunt Ester is a royal pain and so does his mother. And more, the child can feel that his mother doesn't like Aunt Ester either. Now he is getting two messages from his mother that clearly contradict each other. And of course and by far, the strongest message is nonverbal because that is still his predominant means of communication. So when his mother says yes and no and the yes is the strongest, what is there to do but rebel against the no?

He is effectively being told to pretend to be something he is not. Something that, not only is he receiving contradictory messages about, but also goes completely against his nature. He is being told to go against how he feels - against his inherent, real knowing. He strongly wants to be true to himself. His identity is deeply ingrained and it is what he brought with him. He is indeed already being a good little boy by fiercely sticking to the wisdom he was born with.

This battle continues the more his world expands. When they visit Mrs. Jones he goes to her immediately. His mother likes Mrs. Jones and the child is delighted to find another big person that feels a lot like his mother. But Mrs. Smith is a different story. He had always cried when Mrs. Smith held him; and now that he can talk, he lets it be known that he doesn't like Mrs. Smith. And again, he can feel that his mother doesn't like Mrs. Smith either, but he is chastised for expressing his dislike.

And more and more, as he is exposed to the world, he senses something that does not feel right at all. There is a kind of fundamental contradiction coming from a lot of people. To a new member of our world, this opposing information is very glaring. Once he starts tuning into what's really going on around him, he finds it unacceptable. Something just doesn't add up in the way the world seems to be. He can feel something that just isn't natural.

So, as his awareness of what is being demanded of him increases, his rebellion can only increase. He has the formidable force of the truth of the universe behind him which is impossible to deny. He must defend his position or invalidate his very sense of being. So it isn't long before the main word in the child's vocabulary is no. Now we're hearing no at every turn. It gets to the point where the child is effectively saying no to everything. No has become an automatic response. The child seems to take a stance that is in opposition to just about everything he is told. Now he will even say no to common sense and about the things that are for his safety. He flatly refuses to accept the world he has found himself in. The battle lines are clearly drawn.

But of course, he has retained the belief that the big people around him can make it better. So we are still at an impasse. It never occurs to him that his parents cannot fix this problem. They are the gods of this world and have the almighty power. Whatever has gone wrong will be fixed just like before when he had discomfort and he made a noise and the problem was attended to. But no, that's not what happens. Instead, this is when his parents do just the opposite. This is where they really put the pressure on. They become fearful that the child will not adapt properly – this is the critical point where the child starts to lose the battle. Having not yet lost his sensitivity to other forms of communication, he picks up on his parent's fear.

He is starting to make the great transition to this world. He has been introduced to fear.

Once he starts to adopt even just a little bit of that fear, it can only escalate until he starts to conform. He comes to the same conclusion as all those before him: You have to pretend. You have to make believe or nobody will like you. And with constant insistence toward him to that end, he will try it on. Or he may be forced to say something he doesn't want to. One way or another, the first time he acts or says something consistent with what is being demanded of him, he will get strong approval for it. And right there, he has lost his first battle. And it will happen again. Parents, older siblings, and even Aunt Ester will approve and reinforce this preferred behaviour. Everyone around him will strongly indicate, implicitly and explicitly, what the 'proper' conduct is and that this conduct is a matter of grave importance.

After a while, he will begin to doubt himself. He will entertain the possibility that he could be wrong. And he will come to believe that what he feels about himself is wrong and that he must pretend to be what he is being told to be. With the constant influence to conform and with the approval when he does, it's just a matter of time and he has lost the war. Little by little he will forget like everyone else.

He will lose touch with that original wisdom that was meant to serve him so easily and with perfect accuracy. He will forget his very own Divine wisdom that he was born with - that wisdom that is meant to guide him with every choice. Indeed it was guiding him truthfully until he was forced to ignore it.

The admission fee is high for participation in this world. Most people pay because there seems to be no other choice. We must adopt a fictitious sense of self to function in this world. It takes a year or so but most of us gradually conform until we have completely redefined ourselves. We must abandon our true selves - or be abandoned to play on this stage.

Therefore, the rebellion process is critically important so that the child can grow up to function as a 'normal' adult. The child had been fighting a battle that he could not afford to win. That rebellion process is the initiation into this world. We can't function well without going through this experience. We must learn to conform to this world to function in this world.

The age two crisis is critically important and it is how we get the game plan going. For most people, the stage is set at this point. We have conformed to the world. We have created a fictitious sense of self so that we can live in this fictitious world. We have reached the point at which we and reality diverge - until death do we reunite.

But what if it could be different? What would happen if we could again be privy to that innate wisdom we lost? How would the world be different if we were able to use our innate wisdom to contribute to the world? What would happen if we keep our original knowing and take it with us into adulthood? Or what if we could communicate with a child who did not conform and who therefore still had some connection to his inherent knowing?

What we need is a child's mind that has been kept intact into adulthood so that the child has at least some maturity that might allow that original inherent knowing to be expressed. We need a special condition where a child's original knowing was somehow preserved into the later years with at least some ability to function as an adult.

Some children do not rebel for various reasons and with varying results; and they, therefore, will retain their innate wisdom even though it is of no use to them. Some children find themselves in a nonsupporting or even a hostile environment and withdraw. This child is so focused on survival that no development takes place. This child does not take on the world at all. In those kinds of situations, a child never learns and can be dysfunctional to the point of mental illness. The ratio of fear is so great that the child lives in a very shallow world, completely dominated by fear.

So what we need is a delicate balance where a child has kept the original knowing, and yet has been able to become at least semi-functional in the everyday world. Too much withdrawal leads to a dark world, and not enough withdrawal is conformity. What we are looking for is almost a contradiction in terms - a situation that escapes the dark world of complete withdrawal but also escapes conformity. We need someone who withdrew but not so far as to shut the world off completely - someone who withdrew even though he was in a safe environment. Perhaps we need a unique situation where the withdrawal was caused by an outside influence or trauma so that we have cause, but we also have loving support. If we can add a lifetime of experience with partial engagement in life, such a child may very well experience a history of seeing life from a very different view.

Of course, this child will be at least partially dysfunctional. For convenience, we could even use a label to differentiate him from what we call normal. He certainly will be extremely withdrawn. So he might be diagnosed as being mildly autistic or even as having one of the lesser forms of schizophrenia. So let's borrow these terms and refer to our child as autophrenic - an extremely benevolent autophrenic of course. For purposes of this book, an autophrenic is a person still connected to Source and is quite naturally disposed to sharing wisdom from Source.

We are looking for a circumstance in which there is a major change in the outer world of a child at that critical two-year-old juncture so that all the conditions are just right to create a very precise framework. What we need is something like a change in country, culture, and language at the exact time when a two-year-old starts to take on the world. This way, we have a world that suddenly becomes so completely foreign to the child that he does not even get a beginning of an understanding of it to suggest that there was anything to rebel against. The change in language would be the biggest factor, so let's have that huge bridge to the outer world taken away just when a child starts making use of it. The timing would be such that nothing would make sense to this child. He will retreat from this new environment, guaranteed. But he will grow up secure because of the loving home environment. He won't take on the world, but his parents, not understanding what has taken place, will be all the more caring because of the disorder - the perfect framework so that the child will not conform but will engage the world in limited terms. He will retain most of his innate knowing because of that base of a secure and loving environment. Not taking on the world to any great degree, he will have won the battle that we must not win, by default. He will not be indoctrinated into the ways of the world.

Indeed there is such a child. That child exists within each of us. But the important difference with the adult child in our above-created situation is that he may now be able to put a small amount of his original knowing into words; though words cannot possibly fully express inherent knowing.

And somewhere through a lifetime of searching, he may stumble upon scriptures that come close.

Close to explaining the process of *'Retrieving our inherent wisdom'*.

PROLOGUE

And seeing the multitudes, he went up into a mountain: and when he was set, his disciples came unto him: And he opened his mouth, and taught them, saying

I recently had to do a little shopping for a few items that I don't buy every week. Things like soap and other toiletries. I went to a big discount store where they handle these kinds of things. I had never been there, but I was doing not bad, finding just about everything I wanted - until I started looking for razor blades.

I found the aisle without too much difficulty but couldn't find the particular blades that I use. After some time searching, I finally saw them on the highest shelf. Not only were they behind glass, but there was also no visible way of getting them out. Then I noticed a keyhole on the glass that suggested the glass enclosure hinged down when opened with a key. I naturally assumed that these particular items were kept inaccessible for some reason. I knew they were expensive so I thought they were being protected against theft.

I had the good fortune of finding an attendant who helped me out by pulling out a package with some sort of sleight of hand. The blades were accessible after all! The attendant explained that the lock was for the removal of the panel to fill the dispenser. I hadn't noticed that the blades were easily accessible to customers from the bottom of the dispenser. Anyway, the kind clerk removed what I wanted with some tricky little maneuver that I'm sure would have been beyond me even if I had considered this access from the bottom a possibility. It required a certain little twist of the wrist or something. I would have probably had to hold my face just right too. I don't know.

I often find myself in a strange world where these ordinary things of life do not work for me, so I do what I can to safeguard myself from these sorts of ordeals. Normally I would go to a store where things are more expensive but at least accessible. But I was having a very good day and I sort of forgot myself and I took on this challenge and got in over my head. I should have known better. But there I was, once again with some annoying little thing that stopped me cold. And even though the attendant did help me, she looked at me most strangely, as if she imagined that my I.Q. barely registered on the scale. She is right about that. Certain things in this world do indeed defy my abilities.

One would think that I might observe how the clerk had accomplished this little trick of removing the razor blades so that I might have the ability for future reference. But no, that doesn't work either. I've tried this learning thing for these strange little riddles, but there are ever new and mysterious ways of doing things for me to solve. And the advent of the new far exceeds my ability to memorize any useful method. It's quite conceivable that there would be a new puzzle created as often as I need new razor blades.

So, I'm just going to forget about ever understanding how the 'simple' mechanisms of this world work. It's way too frustrating and my success rate is so low that it's just not reasonable to expect that I will ever develop any skills in this area. But I don't really mind. I get by with a little help here and there. The normal way this world functions will just have to remain a mystery to me.

Things work very well in my imaginary world. I imagine that I understand the big mysteries of life. And more, I imagine that I am very proficient at passing this knowledge on. I wouldn't be without that inner world for anything, even if I end up having to grow a beard. And the nice thing about living in an imaginary world is that there is none of this frustrating lack of results that I find my outer world plagued with. And too, there have been times when my imagination bore fruit.

For example, I have always imagined that I could teach. I am told that we teach what we most want to learn. I can believe that. With the tiny bit of teaching that I have done, I have noticed that I learned in the process. And it could very well be that many people who teach have a similar experience. It seems like a good arrangement to me. If that's what it takes to learn, and if those who are the recipients of such activities happen to learn a little as well, it's all to the good. The blind leading the blind is a start if there is nobody around who can see.

What is it like to teach when you already know - when you inherently know and you have nothing to gain for yourself and your only motivation is Love? That must be a whole new ball game when there is no chance or even a desire for any kind of personal gain because nothing is needed. I wonder what that's like. I can't quite get my mind around that in this needy world. And I would venture to guess that that's quite a stretch for a lot of us. A real feeling of all-encompassing unconditional Love for everyone at all times is not something that seems to come naturally in our world.

But what if we could? What if we could find that within ourselves? What would that be like? What would it be like to have all our needs always fulfilled - to need nothing and to therefore be left only with the desire to express Love? The information I have spells out in the plainest language that we - each and every one of us - do indeed have such potential within us:

What I do, ye shall do and greater things shall ye do.

My imagination confirms this. Not only do we have this potential, but it is also our very nature just waiting to emerge. And more, that potential once expressed is what joins heaven and earth.

As things stand now, we don't have terms of reference to understand the great benevolence that sustains us and of which we are a part. But that's what we are trying to fix. It only requires that we patiently release all that we are not. This requires a different approach, leading to a different definition of life.

To him that has it shall be given but to him that has not, even that which he has shall be taken away.

That was in answer to the question: *'Why doth thou speak in parables?*

The beauty of this reply is that even with a direct question on the topic, He still doesn't give a straight answer. But I do. That's what I'm doing here. What has ever been implicit is becoming more and more explicit. And I am part of that process. There are those of us who feel compelled to explain for those who have been too busy trying to keep our world functional.

The significance of that classic answer and its implicit truth is that it is teaching at its best. The teacher insists that you think to understand. Therefore it is far better left alone, and if at any point you feel like leaving my words and staying with the original to get meaning, who could quarrel with that? But assuming my humble efforts have some value, and also assuming that some of these old words could use a little modernizing, I have taken on the task of making the implicit a little more explicit. Starting with the above quote as a sample and because it so beautifully makes my point.

What that quote means is that there can be no learning unless one puts one's brain in gear. We are required to think. I know a lot of us have gotten out of the habit in our automated homogenized world where even culture is pre-cooked and ready to pop in the microwave, but that terrible and contagious affliction of forfeiting our ability to think is literally deadly.

But to him that hath retained or regained the God-given ability to think, all will be given.

So where do we start? With physical things we always have something else to compare to, relate to, build from, or otherwise have a starting point from which to learn. Not so with abstract matters. How do you build on something that you cannot see or be aware of by any of the five senses? We are dealing with inner knowing - degrees of or even the absence thereof.

Probably the best place to start is with the recognition that we are on our own for this endeavour because of our God-given autonomy. Of course, there is always help available to get us back on track. I'm sure there is more than we can imagine in some unseen ways, but when it comes right down to it, we are each responsible for ourselves and nobody can do it for us. It all starts with thinking - pondering and questioning and entertaining the possibility that there might be a better way and that the basic beliefs we have about ourselves might have a tiny flaw or two.

Time out:

I had somebody read what I have written. I needed a little feedback to get some idea of how this might be received. The result was quite favourable except for chapter one. I was told that it was a bit heavy. I was already aware of that, but I like it the way it is. The biblical quotes from which I derive my inspiration have a very powerful beginning, so I don't see a way to make it easier without taking something away.

I think the feedback is valid and I have taken it to heart. I have made a change. I moved chapter one to the end. It may be easier to understand after reading the rest of the book. The great beauty of this modification is that the book has no ending, acknowledging that the possibilities with the wisdom imparted here are infinite. The last I heard, infinity has no end, so the least I can do is create a framework consistent with the topic at hand.

I don't like endings anyway, so this is a gift to anyone who may share the same feeling.

So, on to page 49.

Chapter Two

UPDATE

*Think not that I am come to destroy the law or the prophets:
I am not come to destroy,
but to fulfill.
For verily I say unto you,
Till heaven and earth pass,
one jot or one title shall in no wise pass from the law,
till all be fulfilled.
Whosoever therefore shall break one of these least commandments,
and shall teach men so,
he shall be called the least in the kingdom of heaven:
but whosoever shall do and teach them,
the same shall be called great in the kingdom of heaven.
For I say unto you,
That except your righteousness shall exceed
the righteousness of the scribes and Pharisees,
ye shall in no case enter into the kingdom of heaven.*

  I bought an old computer about ten years ago. I had no intentions of getting a computer at the time. A word processor was all I needed, but I wanted to learn how to type which necessitated a typing tutorial that required the computer.

  I could have just used the hunt and peck or two-finger method, but I didn't like the idea of having to look at the keyboard. I was intrigued by the concept of watching the words I formed in my mind magically appearing on the screen and I wanted to keep my mind free for creative flow. I imagined that I would get good enough that typing would become automatic and my fingers would obey my thoughts without conscious consideration. I'm told that's possible. It hasn't happened yet. I think it has something to do with male genes or something. I have watched the female of the species engaged in several activities while typing as if typing was like breathing. They must have some magical ability that I do not have. But that's another story that I will get into a little later.

I could have written longhand and had my work typed up, but that wasn't feasible either, because I can't read my handwriting. And how about changes? How people ever wrote without a word processor is beyond me. I have the great luxury of adding a sentence into the middle of a paragraph or deleting and generally rearranging to my heart's content. I can even cause whole paragraphs or more to disappear and reappear in another chapter. Is that not magical?

The tutorial was excellent and made it easy to learn. I did learn to type without looking at my hands but I never accomplished much for speed. After a year of practice, I could barely type 30 words per minute, and my accuracy left something to be desired. That dream of typing automatically was no longer a concept. A little disappointing. But.

But what if there was a better way? I had heard of an alternate keyboard. I always wondered why the keyboard I used wasn't in alphabetical order. The letters are all over the place and without any real pattern that I could see. There had to be a reason for the layout, but I didn't know what it was. So I got curious and I got lucky. My curiosity revealed some very interesting information.

It seems that the keyboard we all use was put together a long, long time ago - probably even before we had cars. The original mechanical typewriters were quite primitive compared to what we have now and the typist had to activate levers connected to an arm that had a letter at the end of it. All the arms had to go through the same narrow passage for the letters to make contact with an ink ribbon against the paper.

But apparently, there was a problem with that slot the arms had to go through. If the arms went through too quickly, or if one followed the other too soon, they would jam against each other causing a stall. So somebody cleverly devised a keyboard to avoid this problem. This keyboard had two purposes. One - to place the letters in a location where it was unlikely that two side-by-side levers would be activated in sequence. Good thinking. These people did what they had to do to make this modern contraption work. But the second necessary thing that had to be done really got my attention. Two – to arrange letters in the most difficult sequence to slow a typist down. Both purposes were to stop the jamming.

Good work guys. You did really well because what you did solved the problem. But what this means to me is that I was right. It isn't just me. My inability to achieve a respectable typing speed was due, at least in part, to the fact that I have been given a deliberate handicap.

Sometimes we have to look and see and check other possibilities. Everything we are doing here is about revamping our consciousness, and that certainly doesn't mean conformity to the things of the world that no longer make any sense.

That's not the end of my typing story. Apparently, I'm not the only one who has stumbled over this and taken exception to this cumbersome keyboard layout. Move up a half a century or more from when the typewriter was invented to 1936 and along comes a man named Dvorak. He and at least one helper decided to make a change and went through a painstaking process to make the letters as convenient as possible. Typewriters had improved enough so that the speed limit could be lifted. But also apparently, the thirties was not a good time to invent anything efficient. The powers that be decided efficiency would cause too much unemployment. The thirties was a dark decade – in case you're not old enough to remember. Other attempts were made to introduce this new keyboard layout, but the Dvorak keyboard never went mainstream.

Let's get back to convenience for a moment. How much more convenient do you suppose this alternative keyboard is? Studies were done which is a story all by itself, so I'll make it short: A typist using Dvorak instead of Qwerty - that's named by the beginning letters on your keyboard - moves 'her' fingers 1/16th the distance for the same amount of typing. And people learn to type in less than 1/3rd the time. Guess what I did when I discovered that? Oh yes, after one year I had to unlearn to type and start all over again. But I had a pleasant surprise. After practicing only one hour a day for two weeks, I had made the switch. I was typing at a snail's pace, but my fingers knew where all the letters were and it wasn't too long before I was back up to my speed. And I'm happy to say that it wasn't too much longer before I surpassed my previous record. I'm not going to get involved in any contests, but we don't need to get into that.

One more thing - let's take a fast move from 1936, pass electric typewriters and get to computers. It's nothing to switch to Dvorak with a computer. Just get into the control panel and two or three clicks with the mouse and your computer is in Dvorak. I've never run across a computer that doesn't have Dvorak capability. Of course, the keyboard is all wrong (all except the a and the m actually), but who cares if you don't look at your fingers anyway. And even that problem can be solved if you like. So why hasn't the whole world made the switch? Why aren't we using a keyboard that is ever so much easier in these modern times? Why are we using a keyboard layout that has been obsolete for approximately one lifetime?

Please, someone, tell me we are living in a sane world so that I may have something to aspire to.

Life means change. I am suggesting we can do a little better even as I struggle with change myself. An example:

My son-in-law gave me his 'old' laptop because it was four years old and he had a newer one. I thought my computer was fine but my children insisted it was 'archaic'. So I gave the new computer a try after my son-in-law transferred all my material for me to get me started. Now you need to know that we are looking at about three model changes here: From somewhere in the eighties past Windows 95, and 98, all the way to 2000. And I might have missed one or two.

I was lost. I just couldn't seem to get this thing working for me, even for the simple things. I found all the new things and the many details to attend to way too distracting and frustrating - not to mention the fact that the keyboard on a laptop isn't anywhere near as convenient as a regular keyboard (Did I mention I have a thing about keyboards?). I couldn't get any work done.

I went so far as entertaining the notion that perhaps my-son-in law did not have my best interest at heart, that there could be a subtle but classic competitive antagonism between us, even though he cheerfully helped me out whenever I had a problem. I persevered for a while but I couldn't maintain love in my heart for this computer - or for my-son-in law. Finally, I decided I didn't need the pain and went back to my old one.

But as usual, fate intervened. It happened that I had to move in the middle of all this and my old computer didn't survive the move. Now that was a shock. I was happily established in my new place, some distance from my son-in-law where we wouldn't have to acknowledge that I wasn't using his computer. I had set up my old computer in anticipation of getting back to my normal routine, but no, there was no life in my old computer. It refused to start at all. I couldn't even play solitaire. Very bad situation. I did nothing for a day. I just assumed that cause and effect had taken a day off or that the universe had a major malfunction for my world to collapse like this. I lost all interest in writing.

But sometime in the new day, it came to me that I could at least try solitaire again. And I did get that going. That consoled me and kept me busy for a little while. But after some time I got tired of that activity and, without even realizing what I was doing, I got to poking around with this new computer again. And for some strange reason, I began to understand some of its functions, and the next thing I knew I was writing again. And more, the next bit of information I ran across was that I could plug a regular keyboard into this thing. And so here I am, happily working with a modern computer even though I got here kicking and screaming the whole way.

I actually like modern technology. I like it a lot, even though I display a lot of evidence to the contrary. I am very impressed with email for example. The advantages are immense that it's hard to compare. The cost of sending email is minuscule compared to the costs of sending mail by post and it moves literally at the speed of light, almost directly to its destination. It doesn't use paper. It's efficient, fast, and easy on the environment. We now refer to the old way of mail as snail mail. How soon we forget the speed at which we move letters by post now compared to the days of steamships and the stagecoach.

Our modern technology is truly wondrous and serves us very well. It just keeps getting better with an ever-increasing ability to perform tasks faster and even more reliably. We still have glitches, but technology is much more reliable than say, twenty years ago. And it's changing so fast that it's hard to keep up with it all. It's all good, but we continually have to spend time getting used to the new. We might complain a little, but we know change is inevitable and ultimately we benefit from it.

Today's technology does not make the technology we had thirty-five years ago wrong. The new is just better - that's all. A good example is the computer that was used on the lunar module that made the final descent to the moon. I'm told a somewhat limiting factor was that the computer was maxed out to handle that job. But the computer I am using right now is so vastly superior to that one in 1969, that it's hard to compare. This little computer in front of me would have handled that lunar module with lots to spare. There was nothing wrong with the computers we had in 1969. That technology got us to the moon! It was amazing!

So it's easy to see what has happened over the years. We just kept improving on what we had. We used what we had for a base of understanding and just kept adding on and we still are. We don't belittle the accomplishments of the past. Rather, we honour them by taking them into account as we learn to improve on them.

Change, growth, and updating mean letting go of the old - old ways, old thinking, and anything that can be improved on. The opposite of that is death. There has to be change in life. Stagnation is death anyway you look at it. Continual updating can be a royal pain, but I'll take royal pain any day compared to the alternative. Living means updating on all levels and on a c ontinuing basis.

The New Testament infers an update but that leaves room for misunderstanding. We don't need more confusion at this stage of the game, so please understand that the quotes we are working with herein are an update. We will make use of the old to enhance the new for orderly and enlightened progress!

But this isn't just any new testament that we are living – I should say update. I prefer the modern word, update. This is the final update - one made crystal clear lest there be misunderstanding.

'I am not come to destroy, but to fulfill'.

Is it any wonder we had a two thousand year lead time? Getting clear on the simple fact that we are updating here is that good start that my father always insisted on. He was right. I have found it to be essential. This is the same as installing a fence post into the ground. If we tamp this first little bit of information into our consciousness firmly, the rest will fall into place. But if we don't tamp this first little part in firmly, no amount of tamping on more information will make our knowing secure.

We are now ready for a complete understanding of ourselves. What we are working with here was implied in earlier information. The main difference between these and previous messages is that this is much more explicit. Fulfilling the law and the prophets is to bring clarification and completion to what was only inferred before.

The new is not meant to invalidate the old. Spiritual laws don't change. But our ability to understand does, and has, and will continue to. It is now possible for anyone who so desires, to gain a complete understanding of spiritual law. And I say now because what we have here is even more relevant to our present-day than it was when it was given. We are certainly in a better position to understand this now than two thousand years ago. We have come a long way, and we are living in a much more progressive time. We are now capable of completing our understanding of spiritual law and therefore of returning to optimum functionality.

The overview we covered in chapter one pointed us in the right direction. The first opening statement was all about having an open mind and that's going to come in real handy with this. To be able to expand on previous understanding does require an open mind. We are going to look at some of the older versions of the explanation of spiritual law and expand on them in the next few chapters before we do anything else.

Therefore and before we go any further, I want to take a little side trip to get clear on some of the old terms we are using here. There has been too much misunderstanding over these terms for too long, and as long as we're updating, it's time to get clear on definitions.

'Heaven' and the **'kingdom of heaven'** is a good place to start. We have, and will be seeing these two a lot. They are kind of primary. We use 'heaven' in everyday language: 'Did you have a good time at the party?' 'Oh yes, it was heavenly.' 'Do you want to go see that violent movie with me?' 'Heavens no!' 'Oh, for heaven's sake, get a grip.' We use the term without conscious consideration.

But what would happen if we did some thinking about what we say without thinking? What would happen if we took some of these things to the conscious level? I mentioned before that thinking is a requirement because it defines being human. Subconsciously, we do know what we are saying. We are saying something very significant. We are referring to the ideal. We do know that heaven is the perfect state from which we draw all things. Heaven makes the distinction between our potential and what we are actually living. And referring to heaven also points out our sense of separation from our source, because we need a term that addresses that seeming separation.

So let's look at **'the kingdom of heaven'**. As I pointed out earlier, our command centre is referred to as a kingdom because the jurisdiction one has over one's mind is absolute. Heaven is not that far away. It's as close as a little bit of understanding. Our consciousness - our command centre - needs to be connected to the Great Command Centre to function normally. It's like hooking into the internet, except that the internet is finite. Therefore, any *attempt* at working in God's terms is some connection to Source and is **'the kingdom of heaven.'**

The *'law and the prophets'* probably needs a little work as well. That's about spiritual law. I have explained that spiritual law is absolute, like the law of gravity. We are studying spiritual law here. It is what we are learning about, learning to understand, and learning to apply. So when we get to a complete understanding of spiritual law/cause, it means that effect becomes predictable. As we complete our knowledge and understanding of spiritual law, we become able to predict or 'prophesies' what we have set forth with cause. That's *'the law and the prophets.'*

The *'Scribes and the Pharisees'* represented the status quo (kind of like QWERTY and the denial of Aunt Ester's undeniable bad breath). It also represents the accepted wisdom of biblical times - the base of understanding from which this update expands. That accepted wisdom had outgrown its usefulness then just as now. Again we have a status quo that is ready for a larger understanding. Our status quo is limiting us and it is what we need to see beyond. So in those terms, the Scribes and the Pharisees still exist within us and represent what we are trying to grow beyond.

I've saved the best for the last, although we may have to do a few touch-ups further along. *'Righteousness'* definitely needs some work. It is one of those that have been abused until it's getting hard to recognize. So first, what it is not - Morality. None of this is about morality. We are coming up to an area two chapters from now where it would seem that morality is stirred into the mix, but I assure you that there is absolutely none in this stew. We can confuse the issue easily enough without that. The trouble with morality is that it is defined within normal human activity and that's just exactly what we are endeavouring to go beyond. Morality is usually defined as something one person doesn't want or thinks someone else should do. But that's not what we are doing here. This is about what works.

Righteousness is about understanding spiritual law and the correct application thereof. I mentioned before that it means getting it right, and that's true, but I want to expand that definition now. Righteousness means the right use of The Creative Force / Universal Energy / Love Force. God creates through Love, and as children of God, that's what we are learning to do. I have it on good authority that righteousness in modern language would be right-use-ness - the right use of the God force that an apprentice needs to know about. We use God's energy all the time. There is no other energy to use. This whole thing is about learning to use it right so that we can become functional. Therefore, and incidentally, for anybody who is still interested or concerned about morality, be it known that morality is a result and one of the natural by-products of righteousness.

And while I am defining, I would like it known that I will not be using big words in my explanations, mostly because I don't know any. But aside from that, as we learn more and more about how things work, we eventually come to simplicity. There is absolute simplicity in the workings of the universe. Complicating things is just what we are trying to get away from.

But having said that, there are times when there is only one word that fits, like the word autonomy. That's a word that we need and which we don't need any misunderstanding about. I've already used it a few times and I will be using it again. It's one of my favourites and I can't do without it.

We have reached a point of collective maturity that allows for conclusive understanding. This is a representation of the final dispensation of universal wisdom for those who wish to conform to spiritual law and graduate, after which we will no longer deal in terms of heaven and earth. *'Till heaven and earth pass'.* Heaven and earth will no longer be terms we use to describe where we are and where we are not, because only heaven will exist on earth.

And the cause of the manifestation of heaven on earth will be our complete comprehension and adherence to spiritual law down to the most minute, and exacting detail: *'one jot or one title shall in no wise pass from the law, till all be fulfilled'.* Spiritual laws can't be changed - but we can. When we complete the changes advocated here, we will be expressing our true nature.

Heaven on earth? Don't blame me for being dramatic or too far out there. When He says 'verily', you know something earth-shattering is coming down. I'm not making this up. I'm just reading what's in front of me and putting it into modern language. It's time to be as explicit as possible. As I already pointed out, it's too late in the day for more misunderstanding.

In the meantime, we've got things to do and we've come to a therefore. I think this is the first. I make a big thing about a therefore. Understanding the therefore is of the first importance. The conclusion after an instruction has to make sense or else of course we need to go back and do a little more work until we get it. Or question the credibility of this source. I prefer the former. Therefore, I will be taking special note of this and every future therefore. And since this is our first, I'm sure it's safe to assume that getting clear on this one is essential to that good start that I never get tired of insisting on.

Whosoever therefore shall break one of these least commandments,
and shall teach men so,
he shall be called the least in the kingdom of heaven:
but whosoever shall do and teach them,
the same shall be called great in the kingdom of heaven.
For I say unto you,
That except your righteousness shall exceed
the righteousness of the scribes and Pharisees,
ye shall in no case enter into the kingdom of heaven.

We have established that the old information was just as valid as the new, only less explicit. The meaning was always there for anybody capable of going all the way with it. Granted, that would be a bit of a stretch. But the interpretation of law and our understanding and the practices of the past were the best we could do at the time. Therefore, to invalidate the old and to be a living proponent thereof is a major misunderstanding. That interpretation misses the whole point of these entire instructions and is also a misunderstanding of that which has been given previously. An update works with what has already been established and improves on it. So of course that means understanding what has been already established or how can we improve on it? In other words, a close look at the old reveals the new - implicit in the nature of the old.

Therefore, to be an advocate of the invalidation of the old is the misunderstanding of misunderstandings. Anyone starting with that premise cannot possibly progress towards the completion, understanding, and application of spiritual law. That would be working without a base: *'the least in the kingdom of heaven'*. So it's worth whatever it takes to get the concept here. To discredit old teachings and old ways can only come from a misunderstanding of those old teachings.

But let us quickly acknowledge that we will under no circumstances criticize ourselves for misunderstandings of the past. Or even for the present, or the future. Making mistakes is to be expected and impossible to avoid. We are children learning the lessons of our ultimate potential. We are cared for and cherished more than we can imagine during this process.

So back to misunderstanding:

This is where that open mind is imperative. The ability to take a whole new look at everything and start fresh is essential. Otherwise, it's like following assembly instructions after missing the first line. We could be out of step all the way and then wonder why it didn't come together. There is more to an open mind than just being open to the new. An open mind also means being open to letting go of whatever needs letting go.

We have defined the kingdom of heaven as a relationship with God - working in God's terms. So notice that **'the least in the kingdom of heaven'** doesn't mean that anyone making the mistake pointed out above is less than anybody else. It just indicates a misunderstanding that greatly inhibits progress, that's all. We are in a relationship with God at all levels of understanding. Any awareness and attempt to work in God's terms qualifies your kingdom as the kingdom of heaven.

So there is a key to real progress involved with all this: **but whosoever shall do and teach them, the same shall be called great in the kingdom of heaven:** The only reasonable thing to do is to operate at the level of your understanding. I know that's an 'of course', but there is a bit of tricky ground here. The key to staying out of the quicksand involves doing. It is not possible to go from one step to another without the actual doing of each step before looking to the next. Putting what we know into practice is essential before there can be any consideration of progress. Practicing what we know and where we are is an example and an influence. That's the doing and the teaching. That's working at our finest – working from the terms of our real selves.

And here's the kicker to bring this point to a final conclusion. It's an add-on and a summing up just to make sure there is no misunderstanding: An attempt at new understanding without the actual practice of present understanding has no value at all.

'For I say unto you, that except your righteousness shall exceed the righteousness of the scribes and Pharisees, ye shall in no case enter into the kingdom of heaven.'

These instructions are plain and precise and there is usually one word in the stronger statements that is pivotal to understanding. We have one here that is key to this conclusion and to this entire opening. That word is 'shall'. Shall is a word used to refer to the future and here it means to be in a place where the future holds promise of growth. Shall exceed is to be in a position where our understanding can expand to greater understanding, to where it *shall* exceed the righteousness of the past. Without that, we are regressing; **'*ye shall in no case enter into the kingdom of heaven.*'** That's why somebody at a 'low' level but actually putting that level of knowing into practice is miles ahead of somebody who is at a 'high' level but not putting that knowing into practice. That so-called 'high' level is just information or head knowledge. We need it because it's the starting point, but it's worse than useless until it is integrated, by doing.

I realize that the above statements are very elementary and sort of go without saying. It's easy to understand the principle of learning one thing before taking the next step in learning when it comes to the ordinary things of life. But I have noticed that this simple wisdom is often overlooked when it comes to matters of spirit. There is a reason for this that I would like to explain.

It has to do with the nature of this subject. The business of learning about spirit is in a special category because it has to do with how we define ourselves. It is worthy of all the respect we can muster.

There is a pitfall just made to catch us in this present stage of our development. It's hard to avoid and hard to describe and it can be hard to understand. So put your brain on maximum power for this one - maybe even save it for the morning. Better still, read outdoors. I recommend that highly. I recommend reading out of doors whenever possible because it at least doubles your ability to comprehend.

But here is the pitfall:

One look at the Beatitudes for example and you can easily see how effective that mindset would be, so you immediately adopt it and that's the end of the problem. Or so it seems. Oh, I see, we say, sure, I can do that and away we go. But that's the pitfall. There has to be a process. And yet it's so easy to imagine that you already have what is being suggested here because it feels right and it is your natural home. It rings true and we think we have it. But years of other data and activities of the mind have the momentum and the power and the programming. And more important, all that we have established in the past has the emotional attachment by which we identify ourselves. Those old programs will be the very ones who insist that you have the new mindset established, in order to protect those same old programs. And again, that's the pitfall. It is made in order to trip us up in our present state of consciousness because it is made to order *by* our present state of consciousness.

Let me repeat this in an enlarged version as part of my respect for this topic: We can fall prey to the belief that we have accepted, integrated, and become this information with the first exposure for two reasons. First, we do already know all this - that's the knowing we were born with and does not require words. Deep down somewhere, we are aware of the real truth of our beings. So, when we are exposed to these truths, there is a kind of familiarity to it all that we just accept without further adieu and we disregard the simple fact that we have a huge database within our consciousness that is quite contrary to this. That can stop further learning cold right there. But there's more. The other reason we believe we have this at first glance is that the false beliefs we have developed are threatened by these newcomers. (Yes, we already covered this topic and I'm still covering it because it is pivotal to any real progress!) When new patterns and beliefs threaten old patterns and beliefs, the old trys to incorporate the new to maintain order. If that can't be done because of incompatibility, the old patterns will do whatever is necessary to stay alive, believing that it is protecting you from contradictory information. Your subconscious is your loyal and faithful servant. And the only way this protection can be accomplished is if the old subconscious pattern informs you that the new has been accepted (Oh yes, your subconscious is fully capable of all this and more. There is so much more to us than we realize). So we're back to where we started; we believe we have this. But that's a lie. It's a lie because it is simply not possible to incorporate anything this monumental without a major overhaul.

So that's why you haven't heard the last of this issue (Well, unless you leave now of course). This issue will come up again because it's all about how we have defined ourselves and how that definition is erroneous and how that false identity doesn't give up without a major struggle.

We are capable of lying to ourselves and of being unaware of that lie indefinitely. We have been doing that ever since we learned to cope in this world. That's why I used so much detail in the beginning to make that clear. We bought the big lie to be able to function in this fictitious world, so lying goes with the territory. And that's why we have a warning here.

Great teachers throughout history have come along with Divine timing. As we have made progress, the right One appeared to give us precisely what we needed to hear, at exactly the right time. This has been going on ever since we took that little detour way back when and decided to do things on our own. We were always given what we could handle at the time. It was always the Truth but because of our limited ability that Truth had to be watered down quite a bit and then sweetened up with every new installment, culminating with this full explanation.

So it might be helpful to realize how far away we got and to acknowledge how much has gone into getting us back on track. We have ignored spiritual law and the source of our being or we wouldn't be in the state we're in. So a little appreciation of what has gone into helping us along the way could put things in perspective. And it can get us pointed in the right direction in our efforts to try to understand and appreciate the magnitude of the entire endeavour. Otherwise, we're working from the wrong way down.

The inclination at the level we are at is to want to start with our beliefs and programs that we think are our knowing, keep that, and add on. That won't work. We're the ones who took the detour. There is no way to get back to the highway other than to acknowledge that we're on a dead-end and go look at the map. We need to try on some other ways. What we have been doing is not working.

But nobody in the higher realms of understanding is criticizing us for getting sidetracked. As I pointed out before, it has been most useful and we've learned things that we couldn't have learned any other way. But it is time to stop and have a look around, or we wouldn't be in the middle of a reality check.

Chapter Three
THINE ADVERSARY

*Ye have heard that it was said by them of old time,
Thou shalt not kill;
and whosoever shall kill shall be in danger of the judgment:
But I say unto you,
That whosoever is angry with his brother without a cause
shall be in danger of the judgment:
and whosoever shall say to his brother, Raca
shall be in danger of the council:
but whosoever shall say Thou fool,
shall be in danger of hell fire.
Therefore if thy bring thy gift to the alter,
and there rememberest that thy brother hath ought against thee:
Leave there thy gift before the alter,
and go thy way;
first be reconciled with thy brother,
and then come and offer thy gift.*

*Agree with thine adversary quickly,
whiles thou art in the way with him;
lest at any time the adversary deliver thee to the judge,
and the judge deliver thee to the officer,
and thou be cast into prison.
Verily I say unto thee,
Thou shalt by no means come out thence,
till thou hast paid the uttermost farthing.*

I look up from my computer and watch my neighbour Tom cruising down the street to his house. Once more, the parking space directly in front of his house is occupied by someone visiting Tom's neighbour, Jerry. And as usual, Tom can't see that the place is occupied until he gets very near, so he has to back up to a blank spot about three cars back. His anger is obvious by the speed and manner of the manoeuvre. He's getting good at backing at high speed if nothing else.

Parking his car directly in front of his house is very important to Tom. I know this and the whole neighbourhood knows it. Jerry is keenly aware of it because he has been the recipient of Tom's wrath over the issue. None of us own the street, but that's not a consideration for Tom. He is unyielding in his insistence on 'his' parking spot. Visitors, who do not know about this, unwittingly become the catalyst to this repetitive drama that Tom plays.

Jerry is the loud one in the neighbourhood but he's a good guy and we mostly tolerate him without too much trouble. Jerry is way too busy talking it up all the time, so he knows absolutely nothing about himself. All I know about Jerry is that he has very little chance at change since all his activity seems to be verbal and directed outwards. Tom puts his brain in gear some of the time and he believes himself to be quite progressive in his thinking. But the normal demands of life keep him too busy to actually make changes within himself. I have known Tom for a long time and we have our chats near the street and occasionally he comes in for short visits. I am aware of what causes him to get so angry, but that's one of the topics that we do not explore in-depth.

Tom spent a big part of his childhood in a foster home. The circumstances there were pretty reasonable but there are a couple of things that bothered him a lot and he has kept that with him to this day. The most important memory of Tom's childhood is that he never had a room to himself. It still comes up in conversations, thirty years later.

On the surface, it looks like I could save Tom a lot of trouble by explaining what is causing him to act in this compulsive manner, but I don't and I won't, for at least three reasons. One is that Tom thinks I don't have all my lights on. Next, if I told him, he wouldn't believe me and it would only confirm his suspicions about me. But neither one of those reasons are important. The main reason I do not, and must not give him an explanation of what keeps him in his self-made prison, is that he has to figure it out for himself. He's already in denial about this, even if the truth is very close to the surface. As I mentioned, he refers to it all the time. So if I were to point out the connection to him, I would be performing a great disservice to my young friend. I promise you, he would feel compelled to defend himself. There is nothing else you can do with a strong emotional attachment like that. It has become part of Tom's identity. And in the act of defending himself, he would drive that denial deeper. Well-meaning 'help' like that can and does have its opposite effect.

But that's pretty small potatoes. There is a bigger point to this. An unhappy or even abusive childhood, and or, the endless list of negative human experiences most people have had, won't change spiritual law in the slightest. Tom can keep that circle going until it wears out his body if he wants to, but the laws that govern the universe will be there for all eternity.

I can promise you that Tom often has flashes of his childhood and the absence of a room of his own when he sees a car in 'his' parking place. But these flashes are so common and so fleeting that Tom doesn't give them any attention anymore, other than to let it upset him, and for using it as fuel for anger. All subconsciously of course, he is actually unaware of the process. He is in a vicious cycle that can only be expressed as hellfire.

Yes hell. Hell is right here on earth. Where in heaven's name did we think it might be? Hell has nothing to do with God. So it can only be here where we have somehow got the crazy notion that we can get along without God - that we can be functional while ignoring the laws that keep the universe running smoothly. Yes it is right here and it's been kept in perpetuity, may I say, for a hell of a while. And because of this indefinite time span, we need a stronger term to define hell, which is hellfire. We set up a cause, for which there is an effect, for which there is a cause, for which there is an effect.............! Hellfire is the experiencing of an undesirable effect from an undesirable cause and the cycle that is kept in perpetuity. That's where the expression 'hellfire everlasting' came from.

There has been a little misunderstanding about hell. There is enough hardship in life without imagining that the results of that hardship are further hardship after we die. That's just some silly notion that somebody dreamed up to have control. Like the threat that was used with children that Santa wouldn't come if they weren't good. It's time to give up such outrageous notions. That's motivation by fear. What we are learning here is that Love is the real motivator of all things. That punishment after death thing is getting a little thin. So, for anyone concerned about that old notion of going to hell after death, maybe we better get straight on that too. I will do this now because this whole death thing is very boring and it takes all I've got just to get on the topic. Why anybody would fear death is beyond me. It's just time out is all it is. Life can be a little trying for some of us and we need a break. Not much changes after you die. You take yourself with you everywhere you go. Big surprise! If we create unpleasant experiences here, which of course we will have programmed into our consciousness, we get to keep those limiting beliefs for as long as we want. The tricky part is that the framework you will find after death is too benevolent to provide any great motivation for change. The real action is here on earth, in our physical bodies. It's a lot easier to do it here on earth, where we have this sharp contrast to work within. But as was pointed out earlier, the jurisdiction we have over ourselves is absolute and not even God will change that.

This takes us back to Tom: He is a good citizen and pays his taxes. Tom is Mr. Normal. He is a kindly man with a good heart who loves and cares for his wife and children. And he's a good neighbour. It's because of all these virtues that his little idiosyncrasy is tolerated, even overlooked. To top it all off, Tom is a Godly man. He reads the bible and goes to church regularly. Tom has something that works. He is doing most of the right things and has no reason to change his life - if you don't count the hell part, which he does not. He only takes on this persona from hell when it comes to this parking spot thing. He feels totally justified in this and it never occurs to him that this behaviour is incongruous with the rest of his life - or that it is having a devastating effect on his body and his life. Hell is not all that bad as we can plainly see, if we ignore it and keep the appropriate attitude. Isn't it amazing what we can get used to with a little justification and disregard? Hell seems quite tolerable, but only because we don't have its opposite for comparison. I'll see what I can do about getting on that subject as we get further along.

Now, it's true that this is a very mild form of hell, but it does qualify on the scale. Of course, there are many situations much, much worse than this. There are probably just about as many forms and levels of hell as there are people on the planet, with the possible exception of a few Saints here and there.

Meanwhile, what should we do about Tom? Well, there is nothing anybody can do. Tom is ruler absolute over his kingdom. None of us are even allowed within the boundaries of the kingdom, let alone affect a change for him. Each of us has a sacred place in our personal consciousness that is inviolate. We influence each other all the time of course - big time even. But when it comes right down to it, every individual is just that, an individual. An individual whose inner sanctum no one can intrude within. The only thing we can do is make changes within our own kingdom. And if it's a change along the lines we're working towards here, then it's a major influence. Love is extremely contagious. That would inspire Tom and he wouldn't even know what hit him.

But for now, Tom is stalled in terms of spiritual growth, and he doesn't know why. Yes, his life is good but he feels that something is not right and he is bothered and puzzled by it. He even has coherent moments when he is suddenly struck by this seeming dichotomy in his life. Why isn't he happier he wonders? He has everything he wants. It never occurs to Tom that this one issue permeates everything he does or feels.

Even though he is unaware of it, there is something that is affecting and infecting everything in Tom's life. His good work is certainly not wasted, but it's not very effective as long as he has something counteracting it. His progress is more or less on hold for as long as he keeps his denial. That's why we made such a big thing about the second Beatitude. Acknowledgment is all-important, even crucial to the beginning of change.

I don't know what Tom's future is, but let's imagine what could quite easily happen given the winds of change blowing through the planet these days. For some reason or for no reason or through reading or spending time alone or even through trauma, let's imagine that Tom begins to entertain a different point of view. He starts to explore and question some of his most basic assumptions. Something has happened that has caused Tom to get involved in some very serious introspection. He starts to see a few things about himself that he doesn't like but he believes in himself. He deals with it and he knows it is okay. He can handle it and he knows he can change. And then one day it happens. He starts thinking about 'his' parking place in a slightly different way. At first, he rejects this. Nothing will make him change his mind about that. But it keeps popping up in his mind until he wishes he had never started this introspection thing. Finally, because this issue will not allow him any peace, he decides to look at it full in the face and from every angle.

He's hooked now, there is no going back; it's too late for that. And every time he thinks about 'his' parking place there is another fleeting thought in the back of his mind. Finally, there comes a time when he decides to give that peripheral thought more attention. This thing is getting to him. Bang! It's the old no room to himself memory. He makes the connection, consciously. And, luckily, he's alone because the tears are unstoppable. Tom is in full mourning. The power is too strong. He has to give in to the emotion and the tears continue to flow along with the memory and everything that ever got attached to it. And it gets stronger and stronger until it's almost unbearable. And then it all stops and he wonders how this could have overwhelmed him like that. It's a little scary but he is also starting to feel something new. There is a certain relief seeping into his feelings.

After that the rest is easy. He knows he must reconcile with Jerry. But he's been in this whole process for many months now, so he has also come to realize the importance of keeping new ideas to himself. He wisely decides to put off running over to Jerry's place and explaining it all to him. After a few days, he sees that talking to Jerry is not the right thing to do at all. This whole thing has nothing to do with Jerry. It's all about him, Tom. He now knows to reconcile and make peace with Jerry in his mind, and he does that. Tom knows that the best thing he can do for Jerry is what he just did. His change will be whatever influence on Jerry that Jerry himself decides on.

Shortly after that, Tom has a very pleasant surprise. This issue seems to be settled and he continues with the practices he has adopted. Now, as he works with the ideas that have changed his heart, suddenly there is no resistance within himself - no opposite thoughts clamouring for his attention. He has a certain feeling of peace that he doesn't remember ever having before.

I'm going to leave Tom right there; except to say that it isn't over yet. Tom will have other times of struggle and doubt, but there is no stopping him now.

We each have varying degrees of Tom and Jerry within ourselves and we are each capable of making peace within ourselves. We are capable of freeing ourselves from any and all limitations because of what we are and because we are the ones who adopted those limitations.

The way to freedom is no big secret. It's been around for a while and everything we have ever needed to know has always been forthcoming. The only teensy little glitch is the simple fact that our free will is a two-way street. As much as we are free to do great things, we are also free to forget our true identity and ignore the common sense implicit in the laws of the universe. Our free will makes it impossible for the truth to be imposed upon us. We have to decide that on our own.

Moses freed his people from slavery but there is a little more to the story than that. Those people asked for help. When that request was strong enough and sincere enough and with enough of the people participating in the request, help was forthcoming. It was like Divine intervention except that God does not intervene. A great soul answered the call that was made by the collective free will of the people.

Mind you these same people became enslaved again. But it wasn't quite as bad the second time. They became enslaved centuries later but in a different form. The form of slavery that existed when Jesus walked the earth was not as blatant as it was in the time of Moses, but it was there. Being occupied, controlled, and made to pay taxes to a foreign nation is still slavery, even if it was a little less barbaric.

I, for one, appreciate what has been done, because I think we can learn from it. We're getting better. Democracy has appeared in the last few centuries and is increasing rapidly in our present time. With modern communication and information, we have freedoms now that couldn't have been imagined in biblical times. We are getting closer to freedom but we are not yet free even if our present form of slavery is quite tolerable or hardly noticeable.

As long as we are not exercising our free will in conformity with our inherent natures, we are not free. We leave ourselves vulnerable to exploitation when we conform to the nature of those who want to control nature. The only way to peace, harmony, and freedom is to install the characteristics of peace, harmony, and freedom into the constitution of our individual kingdoms. Once that's done, nothing negative can touch us ever again.

Moses introduced spiritual law in an elementary form to the people he freed. Those laws were given according to the ability to understand at that time. The update to those laws was also given according to the ability to understand at the time they were given. Now we are at a place where it is time to get clear on that update. We've got quite a bit going for us this time and I believe we can pull it off. I believe we can take that last step to absolute freedom. Finally, there are quite a few more of the population saying we have to make some changes. And it's not just John Lennon and Gandhi or Martin Luther King and Nelson Mandela who are saying this; there are millions of people now saying *'love ye one another'*, one way or another.

And we've got the past going for us. We can save an endless amount of time and trouble by seeing ourselves in the people of the past. That's why the importance of honouring the past was emphasized in the last chapter. We can only do it different if we see our own mistakes. And our own mistakes, the mistakes we make in our everyday lives, are depicted in the struggles and difficulties of the past. That's the whole point, or why would we need to wallow in the past? This is hindsight used to advantage.

Chapter Four

FOR BETTER OR FOR WORSE

*Ye have heard that it was said by them of old time,
Thou shalt not commit adultery:
But I say unto you,
That whosoever looketh on a woman to lust after her
hath committed adultery with her already in his heart.*

*And if thy right eye offend thee,
pluck it out, and cast it from thee:
for it is profitable for thee
that one of thy members should perish,
and not that thy whole body should be cast into hell.
And if thy right hand offend thee,
cut it off, and cast it from thee:
for it is profitable for thee
that one of thy members should perish,
and not that thy whole body should be cast into hell.*

*It hath been said,
Whosoever shall put away his wife,
let him give her a writing of divorcement:
But I say unto you,
That whosoever shall put away his wife,
saving for the cause of fornication,
causeth her to commit adultery,
and whosoever shall marry her that is divorced,
committeth adultery*

I pride myself in some understanding of how the universe unfolds and I even dare to imagine that I understand the female of the species just a little. But I have my limits. It looks as if my understanding may never be complete no matter what I do. There are certain things I don't think I am supposed to understand. There are some things that no man can understand. For example, I waited an entire generation to answer one of the many mysteries of the opposite sex.

I had taken notice that women always put the dishes in the sink immediately after a meal. I don't mean that they put them there to wash them right away. Rather they store them there and then take them out again later, run the water, and put them back in. Now to a man, this is a great mystery. No man would ever do that. Logic dictates that you could save a step by just leaving the dishes where they are until you're good and ready to do them or until you run out and have to do them. But not if there is a woman around, into the sink go the dishes. No exception, even if it's not her place. I've had it happen many times by a visiting female friend. Even once by someone who was barely a friend actually, just someone who happened to be in my bachelor domicile for some obscure reason. I've broached the subject with the perpetrators of this strange habit on a few occasions with the hope of getting some understanding, but I could never get a straight answer.

I happen to have the great blessing of a daughter. Don't ask me how this happened. It's another of those mysteries. But behold, there is one female in this world who calls me Dad. Of course, daughters are in a different category. So I have the luxury of a female in my life who bestows gifts upon me in terms of answering the big mysteries of what it is to be female.

I waited patiently for an entire generation until this little angel grew up and had a child of her own and her own home. Then I asked her the big question, "Why do women put the dishes in the sink necessitating their removal to put the plug in and run water and put in soap or whatever you do to wash dishes?" Her answer came without the slightest hesitation as if it was common knowledge that every woman knows. Truly every man should have a daughter to help him understand. The answer was simplicity itself. Why didn't I think of that? And here it is: "In case your mother-in-law drops in." Well! Why didn't somebody tell me that, years ago? Think of the trouble it would have saved me. I went through several relationships trying to figure that out. All I can say is that I don't know where I would be without my daughter.

Women and men are indeed different. But our differences are probably best exemplified in how we hang toilet paper. The standard, accepted way to hang toilet paper is to have the end of the paper hanging towards you from the top. Now, because my generation assumed that such domestic issues were within the exclusive jurisdiction of the female, the toilet paper issue was set by the female. And what man in his right mind would argue with that? Let the paper hang where it will! Who cares? But the key phrase here is, 'in his right mind', which of course excludes me. I think I have made it abundantly clear that sanity is not an issue with me. So I do indeed plunge in where angels fear to tread.

Now a man who is inclined to practicality can see an obvious problem with the accepted standard that is similar to the dishes in the sink issue. Common sense and greater practicality dictate that he hold his counsel and gladly suffer the inconvenience, but as I have indicated, all common sense has been recklessly tossed to the wind here. Therefore, let me put it this way: A man who states his opinion on this matter for whatever reason, be it within the terms of sanity or otherwise, might point out the limitations in the accepted way of hanging toilet paper. He would simply point out that when reaching for toilet paper, one often has to lean over and that in the process a certain part of his anatomy may come into contact with the porcelain. Since this is a rather unpleasant sensation or at least one that most of us would rather not experience, the manoeuvre requires the use of one hand to avoid making the unwanted contact.

Now, none of this would matter if we had three hands. But for some reason the good Lord has seen fit to create us with only two. Of course, God might have considered creating men with three hands and women with two and then thought better of it. Maybe He got concerned that without that female connection to Him, men would be just dumb enough to imagine that they are superior to women if He made us that much different. So He decided to stick with plan A, and let us figure it out for ourselves. His thinking probably was that having created people complete with all His attributes and abilities, we need the challenge. Surely they will see the advantage of putting their differences to good use and find a way that will work for everybody was probably the thinking behind our makeup. So that's how we ended up more or less equal.

But it does require two hands to rip off a chunk of toilet paper when the role is hanging in the accepted manner. If the toilet paper was hung the other way around, one could quite easily put the back of one's hand against the wall, fasten the toilet paper between fingers and thumb and accomplish with one hand what requires two with the accepted way.

So all of this brings us to a key issue: The great and wonderful fact that the male and female have different anatomies. It's all so simple really. All we have to do is become more aware of our differences and celebrate those differences rather than using them as a means for a quarrel, and what wondrous things might we then accomplish. I am absolutely convinced that most women would gladly accommodate us men were they to become acquainted with the problem we encounter with this tissue issue. And more, I know that most of us men would gladly go out of our way in situations where we can be made to understand the different requirements entailed in being female. What man wouldn't gladly put the dishes in the sink when he is made aware of the mother-in-law matter? Or even go as far as to learn to put the toilet seat down.

Still, we could run into some hard going here. But this section is all part of keeping the kingdom tidy and we need to deal with it. So before I take a step into this whole thing about adultery and all these complicated issues of the human condition, I want to offer my apologies to the female of the species. All through this entire thing, we find the word 'he' as if 'she' didn't exist or was somehow secondary. I do the same, but only for convenience. I really don't want to trip over this, or be cute and write things like 'God in her wisdom', although of course, that would be just as accurate and probably more so.

History, looking back at how it was, can be useful for getting a perspective on the likes of *'Thou shalt not commit adultery'*. We can look back to the circumstances that existed when that was handed down to appreciate the difficulties of trying to emerge from darkness. We can have another look at this just like we did with *'Thou shalt not kill'*. As mentioned, they were doing good just to get on topic in those days. You will remember that the people who heard this first had just been released from generations of slavery. It was one of those pivotal moments in history when Divine timing took place and just the right Great One had appeared; there was an openness to something new. That was a long, long time ago but some of us still struggle with that original. That's how powerful an issue this is.

But now, after a new installment on the topic and an additional two thousand years to let it sink in, it could be time to see if we can get the hang of this - to work at getting the full validity and the greater Truth. Is it now possible to come to an understanding of this issue and incorporate this into our consciousness as part of the completion of our reconciliation to spiritual law? In these enlightened times, do we have the ability to make use of this as it was intended without getting bogged down with a bunch of taboos and misunderstanding on the topic? Can we finally understand and make practical use of this information? I think most people would say that the jury is still out on this one. But I think it's worth a try and I think the odds are in our favour.

Again, what was only inferred in the past is now explicit. It's time to understand how things work. That's why it was so important to get started right and get clear on the basics. We have been given a good explanation of cause in our lives, of how the content of our subconscious minds are the determining factor for our conscious thoughts and feelings and how that constitutes the environment in our personal kingdoms, and how that inner environment generates our outer world. So we now have a good understanding of cause. We're picking up the pace here.

The definition of adultery has moved up and been refined along with everything else. The old definition of adultery was sex out of marriage. Now, with the updated explanation of cause we can see what really happens. The simple act of checking shape is adultery when it goes beyond innocent appreciation. Don't blame me for this. I'm not making this up. I'm just reading what's in front of me.

'But I say unto you,
That whosoever looketh on a woman to lust after her
hath committed adultery with her already in his heart.'

That was the easy part. We are coming to some of the heaviest stuff we ever stumble over in this little play we call life. This might not be for everyone. I don't mean that this will be crude. Not even close. I don't do crude. And it's not about morality either. And it's certainly not literal. Take a look above at the suggestions of plucking out your eye or cutting off your hand. I hope that forever clears up what might and might not be literal in the Bible. Does anyone really think that our most loving representative of the Christ would have us mutilate ourselves? Biblical teachings are metaphorical only because there is no other way to approach the topic of spirit. Everything studied is about the one doing the studying. Even the historical references are meant to represent the conditions within the one who would study such matters. That format certainly holds true with what we have here. There is only one topic: The Source of our being and how to reconnect to it. And that includes this part, which is about sex and more, in case you didn't notice. As I said, we're getting into the heavier going here. I won't be offended if you skip this chapter. Trust your feelings on this as in all things.

Checking shape was quite acceptable the last I heard, but it can raise havoc if it gets out of hand. Lust is very powerful and is quite capable of upsetting the balance of the atmosphere in the kingdom. Sex energy is creative life force energy, or how would we be able to create a new life with it? This is the great creative energy at our disposal. It is the energy and intelligence by which creation comes about. So it takes a certain degree of maturity to handle this energy wisely.

In a larger sense, maturity means the ability to co-create with God wisely. We are getting fully on topic here, with an explanation of how to stay out of trouble while we are becoming aware of our defining roles as children of God. Nobody is saying we should have a complete understanding yet, but an outline like we have here sure can be useful. This is an introduction to the nature of the energy we are being invited to use in our job description. We don't have to conform to this of course, but it is the only method that works. As apprentices - children of God - we are trying to learn how God does things.

Any use of Divine energy that is not in harmony with Divine order is adultery. It is to adulterate God's energy. As apprentices, we are expected to make every mistake there is, so that's not a problem. There is absolutely no pressure here. The how-to instructions are here whenever we are ready to make use of them. God's not in a hurry, but I am. I want to get this because I believe this moment in history is here for this very purpose. Reality checks come with Divine timing.

So let's start with puberty because that's when all this starts. Life force energy making itself known at puberty is a much bigger deal than we might assume at first glance. It's a lot more than just an important turning point in our lives. Puberty can be explained and appreciated for the great power that it is rather than taken lightly or ignored. In some cultures, young people are taught how to prepare for this. Rituals and ceremonies acknowledge the significance of this event. In our culture, we are pretty much left to our own devices, and that barnyard learning is usually kept for a lifetime. Is it any wonder we struggle and misunderstand and get ourselves into endless messes in relationships in our western world? Not to mention the fact that we miss the whole point of life: Puberty is the notice that we are co-creators with God in this physical realm.

I've had the great good fortune of meeting some rather unusual people in my life and we need one of them right now. Let me introduce you to Joshua.

Quite a few years ago, while hiking the mountain behind my place, I met Joshua who was thirteen. He was going through a major trauma at the time because his parents had just split up. We got into a conversation over his situation and he gave me the details and explained how and why this was particularly difficult for him. That's when he started to amaze me. His level of maturity, understanding, and ability to discuss his situation was truly astounding. I found myself in a conversation I might expect with someone my age, even though there were almost two generations between us.

This gave me pause and I found myself preoccupied for the rest of the day. I kept getting flashes of this encounter weeks later. Did this really happen? Did I really have a very sophisticated exchange with a child? An exchange that was not only easily on my level, but rather I found my ability challenged at times?

The answer came months later when I chanced to meet Joshua again on my hiking trail. He was in good form with no trace of the unfortunate experience he had been suffering from when we first met. He greeted me like an old friend and once again we got into a most interesting conversation. Only this time it was not personal but rather about the larger questions of life. So I hadn't imagined this grown-up exchange with a child. It was true, he somehow had maturity so far beyond his years that I had no category within which to try to understand this. And more, now I was not able to comprehend everything he talked about. He was treating me as an equal but that was a bit of a stretch. I had to scramble to keep up with him. From there on we had an unspoken agreement that he was the wise one. He effectively became my mentor. Nothing formal - all of our meetings were chance encounters in the mountain.

This brings me to two years later. We have a very firm friendship at this point but limited to the casual and always unexpected visits on the mountain. Sometimes I wouldn't see him for months, but when I did it was always a pleasant surprise. I had been studying the quotes we are working with here and was able to introduce them into our conversations from time to time. On one of these occasions, we had a conversation on the topic we have here, and as always he blew me away with a unique perspective. I have to dig deep into my memory to bring up our conversation but I think it went something like this:

I started, "I just can't wait to hear what you have to say about this. This should be good. I can't tell you how much I've been looking forward to this."

"Sorry to disappoint you, but I think we are going to have to skip this," was the reply, "I don't think I'm qualified for this."

"What!" I exclaimed. I couldn't believe my ears. I had been so looking forward to this and had not bumped into Joshua for a long time. Given the scope of our conversations, it had never occurred to me that there was anything this boy would not discuss. This was unacceptable and I gave voice to my feelings. "You can't be serious. You just come to a tough spot and you decide not to deal with it?"

"There are plenty of other things that are much more worthy of our attention. I assure you," Joshua replied. "I'm sure you can have a great philosophy on life without complicating it with all this. No, I don't think so. You're on your own with this, especially since it seems to mean so much to you. I'm sure you can handle it."

"Oh come on, I can't believe you don't at least have an opinion on this," I insisted.

"How could I possibly understand this?" Joshua replied. "It's all about marriage and grown-up things that adults do. And anyway, you're the adult here. Surely you know more about marriage and adultery and all the rest that goes with it than I do."

"Now isn't this convenient," I laughed. "Are we just going to shift roles whenever you want to? I mean it took me long enough to accept that, somehow, and I still don't know how, you seem to possess knowledge that I do not. And more, I have accepted this outrageous role reversal for lack of a better term. Now you can't have that both ways. What gives here? What am I missing? We've pretty well established that we work on something until we've got it. I don't get this at all," I added with deep disappointment.

"I'm trying to tell you that common sense suggests that you have to be an adult to commit adultery. The very word indicates that," Joshua said quietly.

"What?" I exclaimed. Again I was caught off guard but I thought I saw a way to keep the topic alive. "Is it that simple? Are you just trying to be funny or are you actually suggesting that the word adultery comes from the word adult and somehow is confined to adults?"

"Well yes, I am suggesting something like that." Joshua had a rare smile on his face, even if it was only thin.

I had to ponder that a little. Occasional silences between us had long been established as the norm. I could tell he was serious - as if he was ever anything but. And that little smile only added to his seriousness if anything. Still, I was delighted that we had somehow not abandoned the topic and I wondered where this was going, if anywhere. "O. K., lay it on me," I said with a certain tone of resignation. I knew I was deliberately using that tone of voice dishonestly, pretending that it was me who had been coerced into discussing this but I certainly wasn't beyond a little deception if that's what it took to keep the topic going.

"Well, let's try this on then if you can't leave this thing alone," he said smiling that small smile that indicated he was fully aware of the dynamics between us. "It's probably quite simple if we don't try to complicate it. I think it has to do with maturity, hence the word adult, and or, adultery. A mature person, as in an adult, is expected to act in a mature fashion. If he or she acts without wisdom in regards to sexual energy, then that's adultery. Therefore only an adult can commit adultery. We expect children to be immature, but not adults. And it takes a high degree of maturity and wisdom to handle sexual energy to one's best advantage. There is such a thing as relative maturity among mature people. There, that pretty well explains it, but I'm sure you will want more elaboration."

"Is that all there is to adultery?" I asked.

"Yes," Joshua replied immediately. "And you have asked the right question and that brings us to a major crossroads in common understanding or misunderstanding, I assure you. There has been a huge misunderstanding about this forever and a day."

We were coming up to the forks of the trail where our paths diverged and I could see an analogy coming up. Joshua looked at me with that small smile again. We both got it, but I waited for him to give voice to it. As if he was reading my mind, he said, "yes, this issue is a huge fork on the road for most people."

We said our good-bys, and although we met again, we never did get back on this topic.

Now, these many years later, I understand Joshua and I understand what he was trying to tell me. I don't know if he knew what he was implying back then, but I now see that he had a profound message for me. I cannot deny my own experience. His wisdom, way beyond his years, if not beyond what we might expect in one even of advanced years, is something I had to accept even if common sense told me that this was not possible. I now understand something implicit in his very being back then. I've played it back to myself and it finally makes sense.

The emotional trauma that Joshua was going through when we first met was a key factor in the mystery. I was later privy to additional information and came to realize that the magnitude of this child's suffering was considerably greater than I first thought. And that all-consuming experience was the key to forming his outlook at what is a crucial time in life - the dawning of life force energy to a conscious level, puberty. I believe that Joshua was already quite advanced for his years, even at a younger age, but his unique experience, coinciding with the onset of puberty, propelled him into wisdom.

Life force energy comes complete with all knowledge. Therefore, it is possible, with intentional focus, to direct this energy towards anything we wish. It is possible to deliberately activate the mind to what is considered to be genius-level among other things. And this is what Joshua did, although I believe it was accidental on his part. He was so focused on the trauma in his life, that the new emerging energy within his body was directed by that focus rather than where it might have been. The life force energy, that Divine creative power, was directed to his mind. His amazing wisdom was the result of a natural ability combined with what is normally called a coincidence.

Joshua had an implicit message for me that was more profound than anything with which he had been explicit. His message, implied to me by his very being, was the greatest of all. He was a living example of our greater potential. Our potential is so vastly greater than we commonly accept that it is impossible to find common ground for comparison.

And that's why we are saying if. And that's why I had concerns about presenting this information. And that's why I went so far as to suggest that reading this may not be in everyone's best interest. We can only aspire to certain lofty ideals after some extensive work at the levels beyond where most of us are and certainly beyond the level I am exploring here. Only then, can one expect to feel a natural motivation to pull out all the stops in an endeavour to appreciate what we refer to as sexual energy from a little different perspective.

In the meantime, for us common folk, there is another way to make use of this information, but not by meeting it head-on and getting the crazy notion that we can suddenly aspire to the ideals of a Master. The only way this information can be beneficial for most of us is by allowing it to illuminate a larger understanding of what we are dealing with. By seeing the bigger picture we can sort of see why we trip over this so much. We can appreciate why we struggle with this issue and why it has been the leading factor in just about every tragedy in history. When we recognize, acknowledge, and appreciate that we are dealing with the creative force of the universe within our bodies, we can get a little different perspective. It can make it a little easier to approach the subject with respect, and with a desire for knowledge and understanding.

And if thy right eye offend thee,
pluck it out, and cast it from thee:
for it is profitable for thee that one of thy members should perish,
and not that thy whole body should be cast into hell.
And if thy right hand offend thee
cut it off, and cast it from thee:
for it is profitable for thee
that one of thy members should perish,
and not that thy whole body should be cast into hell.

  That little different perspective I mentioned above is the only way these extreme terms can be understood. This is very strong language. These powerful terms are an indication of the dimension of the power at our disposal. Hellfire seemed like a difficult term until we defined it. Then we made sense of it because it gave us a greater understanding of the power and autonomy that is ours. It's the same with these terms of plucking out an eye and cutting off a hand or having the whole body cast into hell. Good thing we got past literal! Let us not allow these terms to scare us, or conversely, to imagine that the severity of the language used precludes any possibility of relevance.

  It's not too hard to imagine how your hand could offend you. Everyone knows what you do with your hand and it is possible to get to a state where one considers a different point of view. The advice is clear: 'If' that's where you're at, 'if' you come to that conclusion, and or awareness, it is worth any amount of trouble to eradicate that mindset. And that same advice holds for anyone who has a conflict within himself over the activity of his eyes: Checking shape when it goes a little beyond innocent appreciation.

Prolonged misuse of our life force energy has a devastating effect on the body. Therefore, the most radical measures - measures that incur major losses - result in a net gain ... *for it is profitable for thee...*

But let's go back and look at that word that I have been highlighting. There is a little word in here that completely changes everything: 'if'. As usual, we have a pivotal word - one small word that makes all the difference. The 'if' was never, is never, and will never be about the Truth of spiritual law of course. Spiritual laws are not iffy. The 'if' pertains to each of us as individuals. The 'if' honours each of us for the particular space we are in. This is a clear indication of the paramount importance of choice and what is appropriate for each of us. What is appropriate for one person can have very unfortunate results for someone else. We, each and every one of us, must function where we are comfortable and where we feel right. We must trust ourselves above all. That's where I got the idea that it might be the better part of wisdom for some to skip this section. That 'if' is there for a reason. Any attempt to do a 'should' with this can only have tragic and disastrous results.

A misguided concept of sublimating sexual energy can have deplorable consequences. Have we not seen enough evidence of this? There has been every kind of sexual abuse there is, and in places where you would never expect it. That's what happens when you don't know what you're doing. We're dealing with rocket fuel. A little caution and common sense could be useful. Sexual energy will not be ignored. It has a life of its own because it is life force energy. It is the energy that got us here and keeps us going. Ignoring this vital energy or handling it without proper understanding is our peril. It's infinitely better to express than to repress sexual energy. No doubt the benefits of achieving the highest human realization and ideals cannot be measured by any standard we now have, but aspiring to the esoteric and or, sainthood, is not something we are doing here. These lofty aspirations we hear about are all very fine and dandy but look at the mess that comes from misunderstanding. The energy that has the mighty power of creation is worthy of respect. Repressing sexual energy is like repressing anger. That's a powder keg that can only lead to disaster.

So, part of the problem with this section is that it scares most of us off. There has been too much misunderstanding around this topic. Not to mention too much ignorance and dishonesty. Maybe it's time we took another look at this. I for one take the information we have here as very valuable to gain vital knowledge and understanding and as a key to our entire endeavour here on this planet.

We are learning to co-create with God. Surely we need to know something about the creative energy within our bodies. There is something of great value here for us common people living an ordinary life. There is information here that is most useful in helping us to run our lives.

For starters, there is a spiritual law involved that's worth looking at if nothing else. It's called the law of Love and it's all-inclusive. It includes harmony and all the other things that keep the universe functional. It's been set up that way to make sure the universe wouldn't collapse. Therefore, if we learn to work in harmony and with Love, simple reason tells me that we could become functional, which is about as far as I can go with this topic without looking at marriage.

It hath been said,
Whosoever shall put away his wife,
let him give her a writing of divorcement:
But I say unto you,
That whosoever shall put away his wife,
saving for the cause of fornication,
causeth her to commit adultery,
and whosoever shall marry her that is divorced

committeth adultery.

Let's take a little break and go visit Jack and Jill*, to help us through this and see how marriage works or doesn't.

Jack is the one who fell down and hurt his head when he and Jill were going up a hill to get some water, and Jill fell down right behind him. It wasn't all bad though, because Jill knew right then that the two of them were going to get together someday. And sure enough, they dated all through high school and got married when they were both twenty and promptly had three kids. They did pretty well, but going to Jack's parents for Sunday dinner was a real problem. Jill was starting to dread Sundays because Jack always got into an argument with his dad and it would ruin everything for everybody. It got so bad that Jack would be depressed until Thursday, which didn't leave many days for a normal life.

It was Jack's dad who had sent them for water up that infamous hill all those years before, so it was no wonder Jack couldn't think straight. Any country boy can tell you that you won't find water on top of a hill. Water runs downhill and accumulates in the lowest areas. I watched that happen when I was just little. I don't remember a time when that was a mystery to me. So if your father insists on the opposite, it's going to do something to your head. I didn't make that up. The rhyme says that they went 'up' the hill to get water.

For reasons that I have never understood, that's how things were done in the bad old days. We were fed this kind of stuff and left to figure things out on our own. Is it any wonder that many people became dysfunctional and marriages had not much chance?

Jill tried to make some changes to work on this problem, but Jack just wouldn't hear of it. He just kept going back for more. He told Jill that she was crazy and that if she would just act reasonably toward his father, everything would be okay. Things got so bad that Jack and

Jill were hardly talking to one another and they weren't even sharing the same bed anymore. To solve the problem, Jack had an affair. That didn't work so well. That was a lot like expecting to find water on top of a hill. So Jack and Jill fell down again. But this time it wasn't funny. Divorce hurts a lot more than breaking your crown.

*[I am referring to an old, old nursery rhyme here. I checked with my grandchildren and apparently, it's still around. If memory serves, it goes like this: 'Jack and Jill went up the hill to fetch a pail of water. Jack fell down and broke his crown and Jill came tumbling after.]

That was the past, and that's how to arrive at divorce, adultery, and fornication. But none of them work. Even all three together don't accomplish anything. Divorce doesn't work because you cannot divorce yourself from your own problem. Even if you are unaware of the problem, it's going to follow you around everywhere you go. Adultery, whether by the normal definition as sex out of marriage, or whether the word is used for its full definition as the adulteration of the God force, can't possibly work because that's not how creation works. This leaves us with fornication, and that too has its limits. We've shortened that word up quite a bit, but I don't think it's lost any meaning. Fornication is sex for the sake of sex, which is fine, but we can do better. As we have demonstrated, it's hooked into a much larger consideration.

I've watched these terms change over the years. We used to call sex 'sleeping together' and we still do, but somewhere in the sixties we also started calling it making love. I was very impressed with that. It doesn't change anything but it's a step in the right direction.

Divorce is not a law of spirit but marriage is. Marriage, joining of every conceivable kind, is basic to Love and basic to the laws of spirit. That's what we are trying to do: Get reconnected. I think I've made it clear that I'm not on the morality squad, so I'm not too worried about all the silly things we do while we are playing and learning. Yes, all our shenanigans restrict Love from shining through, but it's not that big of a deal. We are indulged and cared for while we are growing up.

I don't want to get too excited about all this just yet. For sure we can do better in how we get together, but to really get started on these kinds of changes, we have to look at the whole picture. There is a lot more coming up to incorporate into our consciousness that will make it easier to get our relationships into a higher order. So it's best to just leave this where it is for now and get back to it after we have integrated the wisdom implied in the rest of this. Then we can look at this part a little more realistically.

When we begin to see ourselves for what we really are, we will enter into personal relationships with a very different perspective. Once we truly know ourselves, these things that we trip over no longer exist. Once Love is in place, everything takes care of itself. Love takes care of itself in inconceivable ways (much more on this later). Yes, we need this information, but for now, let's use it to inspire us to examine and find out more about ourselves. It wouldn't make a lot of sense to imagine that we could do this the other way around. Change comes from the inside out. First, we change within ourselves and then our outer world changes. Behaviour cannot be forced. Our behaviour, habits, and desires are the result of that which we have adopted within - of how we have defined ourselves. All of the above will make more sense as we start to release our fictitious selves and our real selves begin to come through.

So as part of that process, we may one day decide that what we are trying to accomplish with this entire endeavour can be built into marriage. We might start to look at marriage differently than we have in the past. It could be so much easier if we saw marriage as a place to learn something about the nature of Love and unity and even as a place to learn how everything works. Then we may even declare marriage to be a starting point rather than the arrival of Love. We might call a marriage certificate our enrolment into the school of Love. Graduation would come later after the two of us have released and healed all that was in the way, all that was blocking Love from coming through. Marriage truly is the ideal framework within which to learn about ourselves and within which to allow our true selves to emerge.

Chapter Five

AGREEMENT

Again, ye have heard that it hath been said by them of old time,
Thou shalt not forswear thyself,
but shalt perform unto the Lord thine Oaths:
But I say unto you,
Swear not at all;
neither by heaven; for it is God's throne;
Nor by the earth; for it is his footstool:
neither by Jerusalem: for it is the city of the great King.
Neither shalt thou swear by thy head, because thou canst not make one hair white or black.
But let your communication be, Yea, yea; Nay, nay:
for whosoever is more than these cometh of evil.

Mica dam is a huge earth dam at the northernmost point of the Columbia River in British Colombia. It is what is referred to as a fill dam, meaning that it is made of fill rather than concrete. This also means, among other things, that it takes a lot more material than it would with concrete to make it strong enough. The dam is 800 meters across and 243 meters high. I'm not going to bother doing the math, but given that an earth-fill has to have a slope and that therefore this dam must have a huge base, this is a lot of dirt. When it was finished in 1973 it was the world's highest fill dam. So the job of moving this colossal amount of material required many earth-moving machines working in coordination to get the job done.

I happened to know one of the people who worked as a machine operator on that project and he told me a little bit about the nature of the work. There were so many machines involved that it required a kind of synchronization so that the machines could work together in an orderly manner. All operators were in radio contact so they could be commanded from a central control station and thereby directed to move in harmony with one another. Direction was given so that the operators could make minor adjustments in their speed so they would not be in each other's way. The many machines working together effectively became a giant conveyor belt that could only work well with constant minor adjustments. A very impressive operation and it worked.

I, of course, have always insisted on working on my own with the least possible direction, so my concern is about one's every move being monitored and directed. I made the comment that being told what to do at every turn must have been very unpleasant. My friend agreed, but with a little twist. He said that this constant direction was indeed annoying at first, but that after awhile he began to see that he was a part of something much bigger and that he rather enjoyed the experience.

I was so impressed with his comment that I have never forgotten it. A simple working man - like myself - whose main ambition in life was to set a record in beer consumption on Saturday night saw himself in a very different light that day. And he passed that insight on to me.

There is a great oneness of which each of us is a part. That great oneness is best described as God. That's not the only description but let's use it because it has been around forever and we all have some idea about it. I have also heard the great oneness described as 'All that is'. That says it very well too. We certainly need some way of describing unity because that's the basic understanding required to function as human beings.

The central part of our job description is the understanding that we are one; and therefore, it is essential that we work together. So it doesn't really matter what word or words we use, but it does matter that we understand that working together means agreeing on a common way of doing things. There is an omnipresent common denominator from which to facilitate harmony and we need to be aware of that and to be able to refer to it. God is a good word for that common denominator.

But could it be that this term got shortened up or abbreviated way back when? One of our favourite tricks in modern times is to use the first letter in a few words that is a name for something and make something smart-sounding out of it. So I can't help wonder if that is what happened to the word God. That's a very short word for so much meaning. Could it be that the original was something like 'Great Omnipresent Deity'? I'm not sure what happened, but I intend to continue to use the word God to describe all that is because it's really handy. But that's not to diminish the meaning or to be disrespectful in any way.

We need words to communicate with one another. We put letters together to make a word. In this case a G an O and a D and then we use that word to refer to something we don't really understand and that's all fine. It more or less gets the job done. The only problem is that when we use words to describe anything, we usually describe something in terms of something else.

So what terms of reference do we use to describe God? We can use words like infinite and all kinds of other wonderful things, but that still leaves us without terms of reference with which we are familiar. Therefore, what that means is that we don't know what we are talking about when we talk about God. But we do talk about God all the time. So as a further therefore, the only observation to make with all of this, is that we are definitely dealing with what we have to call the unknown. So for the final therefore, be it known that there is only one worthy activity for children of God at this stage - the pursuit of making known that which is unknown and to make this our defining endeavour.

But I'm not going to look for a new word. I'll stay with the familiar. I like the word and who needs the hassle. So let's stay with it, but let's not be afraid of it. It's just a word. Rather, let us have all reference to God be a reminder of what and who we truly are, of our real selves - even if we're not sure what that is.

Still, I do have a bit of leftover concern about using the word God. My biggest concern is that making reference to God suggests a separation. As in, I am here and God is in heaven. We cannot be separate from God no matter what we do, but we can think, imagine, or otherwise believe that we are separate, and I sure don't want to encourage or perpetuate that. We have felt separate for so long that we need some way of referring to our oneness with God rather than separation. We need some way of including ourselves when we refer to God.

Due to the long historical misunderstanding about our nature, whenever we hear a reference to God it sometimes makes us feel less than what we really are. References to God can perpetuate the very misunderstanding that I'm trying to clear up. So where you see the word God written by me, you may think inclusive. And that means you, me, oneness, everyone, the all, our real nature and infinite potential - that which we are trying to remember and get back to. Each and every one of us is an integral part of God and that's not changeable. That's what I mean by God.

Whether we are making conscious reference to God or not, everything we do, think, or accomplish comes from God. There is nothing that is not of God. There is an all-pervasive force containing all intelligence that we employ with our every breath and our every thought whether we know it or not. Therefore, to get anywhere close to doing what we came here to do, we have to make reference to that force and try to learn something about it. There is nothing else that works. We can choose all we want, and we do indeed have free choice, but anything we choose will be from God, including those choices that are not in sync with Divine harmony.

God is everywhere at once. But to be specific and to think and do something at a particular location and to get things done require delegation. You guessed it. That's us. All we have to do is think like God and then the universe unfolds as it should. That's what we are learning to do. So of course there has to be a common denominator. Of course, we all have to operate with the same understanding or how could anything work out? This means that all we have to do is practice until we have that common denominator integrated so that we do it naturally like breathing, and everything will come out as planned. If this kind of thinking was good enough to build the world's biggest fill dam, it makes you wonder what we might accomplish if we *all* saw ourselves in a little different light.

So let's not make this any harder than it has to be. Our free choice is inviolate. So much so that we can and do make choices outside of the will of God. We do it all of the time. Of course, that doesn't work, but the only good thing about choosing dysfunction is that it proves that our free choice is absolute. Our real purpose is to make choices within what works, within the way the universe is set up, which is in oneness and perfect harmony. Our challenge is to get tuned into reality so that we can make choices that are consistent with our real natures. In other words, it would be nice if we knew what we were doing.

This is where thinking comes in real handy. You will remember that I am a strong advocate of thinking. We've been through this before, but please allow me to repeat and expand on this: We are thinkers. Thinking is what we do. We are the thinking part of the universe. So if we don't think, we miss the whole point of what we are and what we came here to do. That would be bad enough, but when we don't think someone else is usually doing our thinking for us. If we do not exercise our right to stand guard on what we will allow into our minds, if we do not spend time keeping the kingdom tidy by sweeping out all that does not match the standard we aspire to, then the influence of others wins by default.

It is imperative that we think deliberately. That we ponder until our thinking is our own, until what we think comes from within ourselves and is above all, original - especially now with the overwhelming amount of information or misinformation we are being subjected to. Outside influence has become so powerful that putting our brains in gear has become critical. We must question what is commonly accepted. We must question conventional wisdom that isn't all that wise, given the fact that it doesn't work.

We each have a conscious mind. We can be aware that we are aware. We can know that we know and we can shut our thinking right off and tune in to higher intelligence. That might not sound like much, but it's everything. So if we don't make thinking a deliberate conscious act, we give up our main defining characteristic. If we do not exercise our ability to make changes by deliberately taking command of what we entertain in our own minds, we run on automatic, subconsciously as the animals do. The ability to think defines us as humans. Thought is our great connection. And the awareness of our ability to choose our thoughts is our reminder of our ability to create. We're it. We are the salt of the earth and the light of the world. If we don't do it, it doesn't get done.

It's quite a responsibility to be a human, but understanding and taking that responsibility has awesome results. I change my mind and everything around me changes. The cosmic computer is pretty impressive. A spreadsheet used in business gives us just a tiny glimpse of what takes place when you change one item - quite amazing actually. A simple mechanical computer can change everything in the program when one item is changed. But with the cosmic computer, it's not just something within a program that changes. Absolutely everything is affected when one person makes a change. It's too mind-boggling to contemplate, so let's not bother. But it all works and we have the authority to activate this mighty power - that's how we are changing the world.

We are the components who actually do something about the infinite potential of the universe. We are that part of God, individualized, which is taking action. Not only are we taking action but we are the action - we are creation. We are the physical creation even as we create. And that's how we got sidetracked.

Please stay with me for a moment, because there is an extremely important point here. It's worth every bit of trouble it might take to get this, and it could save some very time-consuming misunderstandings.

As we have established, God is everywhere at once and to get something done at a particular location requires delegation which is where we come in. But creating within creation can be very distracting. Only the highest level of God's children would take on such an assignment.

'Ye are Gods, all of you sons of the most high and the scriptures cannot be broken.'

That's what we are and that's what we did and we did get distracted.

We got so focused on creation that we forgot that we need to be focused both ways. When we started this project, we planned to focus on creation and Creator at the same time, simultaneously and continually. We are fully capable of that, but as I said, we got a little sidetracked. We got so enamoured with the painting that we forgot about the Artist.

We forgot our very nature - which is all very fine, but it does miss the whole point of what we came here to do. Not to mention that it causes no end to unnecessary hardship.

Because of the very distracting nature of physical existence, we had to forget about all the details of how it all works when we took on this project. It's just too much to think about if we want to get anything done. That part is O.K., and we can continue like that just fine. What's not O.K. is forgetting our own nature. When we get that back, we won't worry about the details of how creation works. When we remember who we are, we will laugh at our silly concerns about how the universe unfolds. Creation works! All the endless details that need attending to are all being looked after. Don't worry about it! The mechanics of creation is in good hands.

We are on the front lines of creation. We are doing the hard part, so you can be sure that everything we need is being taken care of. Yes, we need to know the essentials. We need to know enough to get by and we certainly need to remind ourselves of the main point of this whole endeavour. But guess what? The basics are surprisingly simple.

You don't need to know how a computer works to operate it. If everyone who wanted to use a computer had to know how it works, nothing would ever get done. There really isn't much to learning how to operate a computer and there isn't much to learning how to activate creation. In both cases, aside from minor instructions, the main thing you need is trust. If you need more, some geniuses know all about computers and some Great Masters know all about how the universe works - that's good enough for me.

Of course, there is a big difference between spirit and our technology, even if there is a similarity. In particular, there is one big difference that can throw us off our present stage of development. Activation is indeed as simple as clicking onto an icon, but there is an automatic fail-safe characteristic built into creation so we don't kill ourselves in the learning process - at least it is hoped that this safeguard will keep the fatalities low. I don't think most of us would be too happy with the results if all of our thoughts became instantly manifested. We are lovingly cared for while we learn. Thankfully, in this stage of our development, our thoughts require repetition to acquire the necessary power to manifest. We have to become familiar with something before we have feeling for it. And feeling is the key. Feeling is the power and our safeguard and also the big holdup. Feeling is the great connecter to all things and how things get done. Feeling is the power because it is energy in motion as in emotion or e-motion. And it is our safeguard and the big holdup because it is usually impossible for us to conjure up strong feeling about anything until we have familiarity with it through repetition. The ability to direct and deploy thought and feeling is our defining activity. So the trick is to do it deliberately and consciously because it works whether we are paying attention or not. If we don't take charge of our thoughts, we create by default - by whatever we *unthinkingly* allow into our minds.

We have touched on this before and we will be looking at this again from every angle I can think of. It is our core issue and our big stumbling block because it has to do with our false identity - that fictitious identity we had to adopt as a requirement to participate in this world of fiction and which we are trying to leave behind and get beyond. We will keep coming back to this issue because it is tricky ground.

Part of the pitfall is that there has to be a process to revamping the kingdom. That process can be tedious and seem uncertain. Because of that, and in that interim, that time span can be misleading. Our old beliefs can take that opportunity to declare that the system doesn't work and we give it up and perpetuate the lie.

We have to learn to use our power. Relearn would describe it better. We have to relearn because we unlearned it during all that time we were busy forgetting what we are. So remembering would describe the process better. Let's remember that we are in the process of remembering. And the day will come when we will be in touch with our real selves again. We will therefore and thereafter, always feel the ultimate feeling and then repetition will no longer be necessary. Yes, most of us have a bit of work to do before we can hold steady to that state, but it's nice to know that Divine Love works instantly. Miracles take a bit of practice and a lot of getting used to.

Those old thought patterns that don't serve us too well took a lot of repetition to become part of the establishment. Feelings for the things we accepted by default was a process, and feeling for anything we desire is a process. The good news is that the positive and loving furnishings of the kingdom to which we are aspiring are much easier to establish. The universe is predisposed to benevolence and the creation of that which is good. By contrast, it sometimes takes a lifetime to create something negative like poor health.

Due to the limitations we imposed on ourselves during our time of forgetfulness, we must be a little cautious about making life-changing decisions. We are not in a position to know what decisions we might make in the future because of the simple fact that we do not really know *ourselves* yet.

There is a warning here about taking oaths and making promises or otherwise mortgaging our future. This is an important bit of information to take along on the road back to remembering the Truth about ourselves. We can't possibly make promises when we don't really know where we are going with all this, at this defining stage of our development. How can we know what we might be doing in the future, given the huge disparity between the narrow definition we have of ourselves and the great truth of what we really are? When we become aware of the truth about ourselves and learn to function on that level, we will be working from a much larger perspective - a perspective that we cannot yet see from the point of view from which we are emerging.

Therefore, declarations about our allegiance, how we will conduct ourselves, and even a definition of ourselves cannot be made within how we presently know ourselves. That would be like a little boy deciding that he will be a fireman when he grows up. He might, but he might not. What if space travel becomes prevalent in the future? Space travel may have been entirely unknown at the time of this child's decision. All these things are good, especially imagination and daydreams. Imagination is healthy and wholesome and a wonderful part of us. Imagination is one of our divine faculties. Where would we be without imagination? But where are we without flexibility? So let's not tie ourselves into something that might be difficult to disengage from. We don't know enough about ourselves yet. Everything is changeable while we are redefining ourselves and finding out how things work. Ways of doing things - or even spiritual practices that may have been in the family for generations - are all up for grabs now.

Blessed are the poor in spirit: for theirs is the kingdom of heaven.

It's important that we be open and flexible to take this final step home. Learning to use power requires a certain maturity and a certain understanding. We have been delegated the use of power but it does not belong to us as individuals. How could it? As has been pointed out, the universe can only work in Divine harmony with a common denominator. We are in the process of learning how to use power in a way that will work in harmony. That's why and how our power is limited. As we learn how to use power in accord with the source of that power, we automatically gain more power because that power wants to be used, it wants to enlarge itself. Creative power wants to create, but it can only work constructively. So as we understand the right use of power, we quite naturally access more power. But for now, there is still a gap between where we are and where we are going. There is still a gap between what we are experiencing and our potential. There is a gap between what we think we are and what we really are.

And the biggest gap - and the big leap to knowing ourselves - is the understanding that we don't create anything at all. We do activate creation. But the potential, the raw material and power with which to create, is already in place. So let me put your mind at rest about power. We don't really have any power whatsoever of our own. *'thou canst not make one hair white or black.'* That should help to put things in perspective. I notice we have no trouble giving our computers credit for what they accomplish. I wonder what would happen if we give credit to the great cosmic computer that runs all things and keeps the universe operating smoothly.

We have adopted the habit of focusing and identifying with what we see. We can see a computer and we can work and play with it and even acknowledge its amazing abilities. But that kind of first-hand evidence is not as readily available when it comes to the operation of the universe. It's easy to overlook and it's easy instead to focus on that which demands our attention. So how do we focus on a force that is so benevolent and unobtrusive that it makes no demands on us whatsoever? How do we focus on this force that supports us unconditionally and quietly in all of our endeavours to the point of being unnoticeable?

Free will: We have only to apply willingness. To exercise our free will is to be will-ing. We have only to be willing to exercise our free will towards going beyond our normal boundaries and to be willing to try to understand.

As we find out a little more about ourselves, we will probably get a little more agreeable. And somewhere along the line, most of us will probably want to agree with the way everything is set up. As we start remembering who we are, we will quite naturally agree with our true nature. Agreement means saying yes. Yes to Divine harmony and no to any suggestion of limitation, and or, negativity. We will in effect, will God's will.

But let your communication be, Yea, yea; Nay, nay: for whosoever is more than these cometh of evil.

There seem to be three things we have to be clear on before we can even start to understand the system. First is Communication. For sure we have to be clear on that. Nothing can take place without communication with our source. Next would be agreement. We can't do much unless we agree with the system, which takes us to number three. Power. Communication and agreement are how we get hooked into our power. So how can we do *'more'* than that? Well of course we can't. But we try to, and that's how we get into trouble. In fact, trying to do *'more'* than that is our whole problem. Trying to do more means trying to work outside of the system. This of course is totally outrageous and absurd. It is how we lose our power. But we will get to that in good time. The folly of our ways is fully covered later. For now, we have this simple statement to get us more on topic and give us something to think about so that we can tie it all together later. We have had a communication breakdown and the repairing thereof is the nature of this endeavour.

So this is, has been, and will continue to be, all about getting reconnected to our power. And our power is all about agreement. Agreement with the only power there is - agreement with the source of our power. Therefore, it is all about communication. And real communication is, quite naturally, communication with the source of our being and our real nature. And it's about the quality of that communication. It's about communication in agreement with our own nature and it's about disagreement with any and all suggestions of limitation from the world - the world we have fabricated in darkness and is inclined to perpetuity if we let it.

Let's flashback to the beginning for a moment, to the part where it was pointed out that we are the salt of the earth and the light of the world - and to the conclusion that if we don't do it, it won't get done. Now it's obvious that to get anything done, we have to agree with the system. We have to agree with how it all works. As mentioned, we agree with our computers; we agree with how they work and make commands according to how they function. So it might help if we agree with the big system.

This is the update on this topic, and in keeping with the nature of this entire update, it is the final word on the matter. It is a big step from what we have previously accepted. In the past, it was necessary to declare some sort of allegiance to get a start on a concept beyond our individual selves. But with greater understanding, that allegiance is understood without saying; it's included within the definition of ourselves. Again, we are not invalidating the old, just clarifying and adding on. Your allegiance is to yourself as part of God. Now that we are ready to learn the truth about ourselves and the truth about how things work, we don't make promises at all, not even to God. Now, rather than making promises, we make an agreement. We are ready to agree with the truth about ourselves and therefore agree with God. We are ready to re-evaluate ourselves, to come to an understanding about ourselves from an entirely different perspective. That's the understanding that effectively redefines us from a narrow sense of identity confined to a body, to our real identity as one part of the Great Self.

Identifying only with the body is a little like having a toothache. A real bad one can demand all your attention to the exclusion of all else. But when you get the tooth fixed or get rid of it or otherwise solve the problem, you can come back to the realization that there is a lot more to you than a tooth.

I don't recommend getting rid of the body, but I do recommend getting rid of that exclusive identity. Also, I have noticed that when we get a cavity filled most of the work the dentist does is in drilling out the part that has decayed. The actual filling doesn't take long at all. And it's the same with this little project we are working on. Getting rid of the part that is causing decay within ourselves, is the bigger job. After that, filling ourselves with the new is quite easy. It happens almost automatically.

Chapter Six

GIVING

*Ye have heard that it hath been said,
An eye for an eye, and a tooth for a tooth:
But I say unto you, That you resist not evil:
but whosoever shall smite thee on thy right cheek,
turn to him the other also.
And if any man will sue thee at the law,
and take away thy coat,
let him have thy cloke also.
And whosoever shall compel thee to go a mile,
go with him twain.
Give to him that asketh thee,
and from him that would borrow of thee turn not thou away.*

I remember learning how to back up a semi-trailer. It was one thing to turn my head around and look back to see what I was doing. With an empty truck that had no sides, I could see everything and learned without much trouble. But with a load on, it was essential that I used the mirrors – now that's a whole new element in learning to back up a semi-trailer. Today there are training courses and many guidelines and regulations, which means that the student is taught the use of mirrors right from the beginning. But that's not how it was when I learned. I started driving without any instruction whatsoever. Jump in and go was the technique at the time. Someone rode with me for a while but he didn't seem to know much more than I did, so I more or less figured out what to do on my own. The good old days indeed. There wasn't even a test. We paid one dollar to get our class 'C' license and started driving. That approach is so unthinkable now that I'm sure this little story is hard to believe. But let's get back to backing up. That's a lot easier than trying to fathom how things were done a half-century ago.

When you back up a car, or a truck without a trailer, it's no big trick because you start your manoeuvre by turning the steering wheel the same way you do when you are going forward. I say start your manoeuvre because to complete the manoeuvre it is necessary to turn the wheel the other way to cancel the turn or you will just go around in circles. Backward or forward with a car requires the same direction of the steering wheel, except when backing up the front end goes in the opposite direction of the required direction to facilitate the directional change of the vehicle.

So let's throw in an additional factor with a semi-trailer - to start the manoeuvre, it is necessary to turn the steering wheel in the opposite direction than the direction you would have the trailer go. Once the directional change has begun, it is necessary to make two additional directional changes with the steering wheel to cancel the directional change and to 'follow' the trailer to the established direction. And more, each further directional change requires the same three directional changes of the steering wheel.

Let's add mirrors. The thing about mirrors, which anyone who has ever looked into one probably knows, is that it shows everything backward. Do you see where I'm going with this? Do you care? This is not an earth-shattering revelation I am sharing with you here but I might have a point. So let's go back to backing up a semi-trailer and the simple but necessary consideration when you add the mirror factor. Since everything is backward in a mirror and we are already turning the 'wrong' way for a semi-trailer, now we have an additional 'wrong' way element to factor in. I hope this is getting extremely complicated otherwise it won't be any fun. With all these factors, one wonders how anybody ever learns to back up a semi-trailer!

Most people, of course, never think about this at all when they are learning. They just do it. They work at it until they have it and that's the end of the matter. Not so for me. It never occurred to me that I could do something without understanding the whole process. I can't tell you how much that slows the learning process down. But when you come into this world and it doesn't seem to work as you expect - and others seem to learn more simply than yourself - what is there to do but try and figure it out? Or say the hell with it.

So back to the semi-trailer: I did things the hard way and ran all the details through my mind to learn. Yet, I had a most pleasant surprise. Since a mirror shows things backward and since it is necessary to turn the opposite way to the direction you want to back up a semi-trailer, guess what? These two factors cancel each other out and we are back to turning as if we had no trailer. I could look in the mirror and pretend there was no mirror and that I did not have a trailer and it worked. At least to get started, before making the additional turns required to cancel and follow. But that's easy because once you get started the other changes become automatic. After turning in one direction, there is only one other choice. There are only two directions that we can turn a steering wheel. Life is so simple when you don't mess with it.

But just in case anyone does not fully appreciate the fine art of making a simple thing complicated, I will throw in one more factor. May I introduce the joy of backing up two trailers - two trailers hooked together by an additional fifth wheel? What we commonly refer to as a B train. Forget the mirror for a moment. One assumes that we are well past translating the mirror effect in our minds when we get to this stage. The combination of trailers we refer to as a B train requires an additional reverse turn of the steering wheel to begin the directional change, which makes a grand total of four directional changes in the steering wheel for each one directional change of the entire vehicle. So, if you ever observe someone backing up a trailer or a combination of trailers and wonder why he is turning the wheel so much, that's the answer. Of course for someone just learning there will be even more turning involved because of the errors made. The difficulty increases exponentially with additional swivel points to the point that to add one more than that of a B train is generally considered impossible. There may be rare exceptions to this, but I'm not one of them.

It's truly amazing how well our subconscious minds serve us! The process of learning/programming our subconscious minds for such a complicated manoeuvre can be slow and tedious, but once it's in there, look what happens. It leaves us completely free on the conscious level - as we are meant to be. I'm no better than anyone else at this, but I can back up a B train while I'm forming the words in my mind of how to explain it all, or while I'm trying to remember a phone number so that I can have a dance partner for Saturday night.

I seldom think about what I see in a mirror, whether it's a trailer, a combination of trailers, or my face when I am shaving. We can get used to just about anything. And apparently, we can get used to seeing everything backwards if we think it serves our purpose. We can get so used to seeing everything backwards that it seems normal.

The word 'live' backward is the word evil. I don't know how that came about, but it sure makes a point. The word evil sounds scary. It's about the strongest term we have for something that is not good. But the word live as in 'live and let live', has an opposite effect. So I don't think we need to be afraid of the word evil, or be afraid of the meaning of the word for that matter. Evil is just getting things backwards anyway you look at it. We can get so used to evil that it almost seems normal. It's just part of our world. And in that seeming normality, it seems quite logical to fight against it, if we have to. It is quite logical to take whatever steps are necessary to protect ourselves. Doing battle with anyone with evil intent towards us is entirely reasonable.

But apparently, that doesn't work. That was part of the old ways, the old ways that we are looking at for updating, understanding, and taking a step beyond. And that step beyond would have us do the opposite. If I've got this right, when someone is doing bad things to me or ripping me off, the suggestion here is that I go out of my way to not only freely allow this, but give him something else besides. It seems to me that this approach is just as radical as the old eye for an eye thing. Why would we do such a thing? It almost seems like we are being asked to give up reason here. Reason is not that big of a deal for me. But what about normal people?

So the update on this *'eye for an eye'* issue, as we can expect by now, is not some minor adjustment. It's more like a complete about-turn. We can make this complicated if we want to, but it is not. It's actually easy. It's as easy as looking ourselves in the mirror. And as before, if we understand the past, we can use it as a base on which to expand. And also as before, the old law was an introduction to cause and effect. It made the point, even if it now seems harsh or archaic. That old law has not changed. What goes around comes around and we do indeed invite into our lives whatever we put out. That's an unchangeable law of the universe. No problem with understanding there. We are well versed about that at this point.

The *'eye for on eye'* was the kind of approach necessary when there was no knowledge of cause and effect. It was and is the truth of how things work. That was and is still valid law, and it is still useful as a reminder of cause and effect. It is essential to understanding. But it is not essential to literally *enact* this spiritual law into our human laws. We have made progress. We can now understand the consequences of our actions without being hit over the head with it. Who would do such a thing to anybody else in the full knowledge of what he is bringing into his own life by an eternal law that cannot fail or be avoided? Understanding cause and effect suggests that we are ready to put a cause into effect that is more in keeping with our nature and has much more favourable consequences. So if somebody wants to involve you in some kind of negative exchange, it is now obvious that it's worth any amount of trouble to avoid it. Who needs the pain?

Therefore the updated way to handle any aggravation coming our way is obvious and simple. Not easy by any means. In fact I would call this a major challenge - maybe even the biggest challenge we could run across while we are trying to find our way. But the only possible way to stop the endless back and forth of disagreeable exchanges of any kind is to agree. This has been implicit and explicit from the start. We saw that in the Beatitudes and again in everything we have looked at so far. And especially in the last chapter where it was made crystal clear that agreement was the name of the game as the way to getting reconnected to power. This part puts agreement to the test.

So let's look at what happens when you do the opposite of that - when you do resist. I don't think we are going to be short of examples for that. Just turn on the television. I can assure you that at the time of this writing there are many present-day examples of the results of someone resisting evil by reciprocating. It certainly seems like a good idea and it certainly seems to be the logical thing to do. The only problem with this logic though, is that it's not working.

It's too bad, but that method doesn't work. And it has never worked, even if it seems like it should. If somebody is very clearly in the wrong by taking something of yours or doing you harm for no reason, well then, you would think saying no or otherwise raising a fuss to let this person know that he is out of line, would do the trick. Reason tells us that the other person will see the error of his ways, especially when we give him back the same or more of the same. And reason tells us also, that he will therefore stop this unreasonable action. So that should be the end of the matter.

But when you are dealing with anybody who has already bypassed, lost, or otherwise overlooked any semblance of real understanding and has therefore also lost the concept of Truth, and that same somebody is confronted with a 'reasonable' reaction, there is going to be a problem. And the problem can only get bigger. Confrontation is fuel for the fire. It only strengthens the unreasonable reason your aggressor has for his actions. It gives him 'reason' to continue his actions. Now he is more justified than ever because you have transgressed against him proving to him that you are the wrong one. Now for sure, he will not look at his own actions.

This business of not looking at one's actions brings up an interesting point: Not looking at our own behaviour does not mean that we are entirely unaware of what we are doing. On the subconscious level, we are quite aware of course. Just like when I back up a B train without any conscious thought, any one of us can be doing almost anything without conscious thought. But that does not mean that there is no awareness. When I am making that complicated backing manoeuvre without any conscious thought, each and every detail of the manoeuvre is being attended to by my subconscious mind. And it's right there, at the periphery of my awareness. I could direct my attention to it with only a slight shift in focus. And likewise, when any of us are very busy defending an indefensible position, we could shift our focus to the greater truth that exists within our subconscious minds.

We do indeed have access to all necessary information at any given moment. But as conscious beings, we focus our attention where we will. And when we are in denial about our behaviour, our focus is of course on anything except that which we are denying so that we can defend the position we have taken. We know full well on the subconscious level when we are not in truth. Therefore, when someone else points out that denial by bringing up that which we wish to ignore, it can only increase that denial - it can only bring about an emotional reaction to defend the position taken.

The point to this is that denial is hard enough to maintain by oneself, so an attack by someone else is actually welcome because it allows one to strengthen the position. The mechanics of all this is on the subconscious level because that's the very nature of denial. But so too does the very nature of our entire problem with the human condition exist on a subconscious level and in denial.

Still, that which we are in denial about is not quite as easy to correct as correcting a directional change with my B train. If I have made an error with backing and I find that the trailers are not going where I want them to, I have to stop and take it to the conscious level to make a correction. And that's precisely what we have to do when our lives are not going where we want, even if it is a little more challenging.

Programming my mind with the ability to back up a B train is software; it is just one of any number of things we can add to the hardware we come with. We come with the basics; we are hardwired with what we need and with the ability to add any software we choose. The basics we come with is our inherent knowing about ourselves - that knowing that we allowed to be overridden at an early age and that we had to forget to function in this fictitious world. Most of us have indeed hidden that knowing from ourselves as directed. But that doesn't mean that that inherent knowing no longer exists. We can ignore our real knowing, but we cannot erase it. It's still there, ever-present and ready to be acknowledged and put to good use whenever we are ready. But that's a personal endeavour that cannot be forced even by ourselves, so it sure can't be forced by someone else and with confrontation (much more on that later).

So, where the bigger problem comes in with confrontation is that it threatens the whole system. When you confront someone by bringing any particular negative behaviour to his attention, you are doing a little more than the obvious. You are touching on the base of the entire belief system that had to be established in order to function in this world. That whole house of cards could come tumbling down if your opponent allows this truth in. And that's why and how you enlist someone's anger with confrontation. Confrontation exposes that which has been established as an *identity*. No one can afford to allow information in that would contradict that hard-earned sense of self. That's why confrontation cannot, and does not work, and can only have the opposite effect. Force cannot, and does not work when it comes to personal change. It is a contradiction in terms. Force works for getting a rocket into space, but force will not change anybody. Only Love can affect a change (and again, much more on that later).

Trying to solve a conflict with conflict cannot work. It is not possible to find out the absolute truth about the many details that led up to a conflict, of how someone came to initiate negative action. No matter how sure we are about being right, we can be just as sure that there is at least one factor that we are unaware of. There has to be, or there would not have been a conflict to start with. All disharmony of any kind comes from something we are unaware of. Our reasons for conflict stem from the limited perspective that we are trying to overcome. And again, that limited perspective cannot be forcibly changed. There is no other way than to just drop it. Drop whatever it is and start over. Give it up, forgive, or have the consequence of disharmony around you indefinitely.

Of course, that doesn't mean that you let yourself be a doormat: Anything but. What this means is that you don't allow yourself to get sucked into a negative exchange to start with. And it means caring about yourself enough to get away and stay away from anyone who does not show any basic understanding about their inappropriate action toward you.

Aside from the fact that a negative reaction to negativity doesn't work - aside from the fact that confronting someone who is transgressing upon you one way or another only enlists further wrath - there is something else to consider. The real problem with this reaction on the part of any of us who is being transgressed upon, is that this approach is in itself a negative activity that can only harm us. It can only put a cause into effect that we do not want. We can be perfectly justified, but that won't change the law or the effect of what we put out. We still put a cause into effect that must come to us no matter what the reason. The law is impartial - it has to be or the system couldn't work.

No doubt all the above is not easy, but that's the way the world is right now and the only way to change it is to start doing something that works. Our world is not currently based on universal truth, but it is the reality that we made up while taking this little time out - while trying to make a go of things without being aware of the laws of the universe or imagining that we could function without being connected to the source of our being. We will not solve our problems within the terms of the fictitious world we created.

The critical factor in all conflict is that which is unknown to us. Each person will be convinced that it is the other one who started it. The problem is that each person is right and each person is wrong. Each person is right because each person bases his truth only on that which he chooses to place his attention on. And each person is wrong for the same reason. But there is a third party involved here who is always ignored: Mr. Misunderstanding is the one who started it. He's the one to blame and the one who should suffer the death penalty. But as long as we have something within us that we have not looked at to release and heal, Mr.

Misunderstanding will be alive and well. As long as we do not really know ourselves, how can there not be misunderstanding? As long as we identify ourselves based on a false premise, there is no telling the particular way that that distortion will show itself in any particular person. And since all of our interaction takes place within this limited understanding of ourselves, there has to be misunderstanding. We are not yet working from that great common denominator that would eliminate any possibility of misunderstanding. Each of us personalizes misunderstanding in our unique way.

So I can only repeat that this comes down to a catch 22 - like it always does. We need to be in touch with our true selves to be able to solve conflict, but conflict keeps us out of touch with our true selves. This turning the other cheek concept is not for your first day at school. That's why we covered the easier stuff first.

We just had a whole chapter on the advantages of being agreeable. Not to mention the fact that just about everything we have covered so far is about being agreeable. So I think it is reasonable to assume that we are not yet finished with this agreeing thing. Being agreeable the way it was described in the last chapter, points out the necessity of agreeing with our true nature. And now we are immediately confronted with what that truly means, with that concept put to the test.

Our true nature is the power because it is hooked into the only real power. So when we stick with that concept under any and all circumstances, everything changes. Resistance doesn't work; we know that. **'Resist not evil'** is the ultimate in being agreeable to our true nature. There was a popular cliché just a few years ago that is probably extinct by now, but made a very good point: 'Don't even go there'. This is just one more way that the truth is seeping in everywhere. It is indeed all around us and in many of our popular sayings.

When someone is being unreasonable and you yield, you present him with a problem. You have taken away his focus. Negativity has no power of its own. It is very dependent on reactive support to stay alive. It has nothing to do with Love and is certainly not Love's opposite. Love stands by itself. So when you comply with an unreasonable request, you have actually taken away fuel for the fire of your opponent's animosity. He cannot focus his animosity towards you because there is none to work against. So now with no opposition and with his focus not quite so unyielding, the fuel that powered his behaviour has been reduced considerably.

That can have an interesting effect. Your opponent will have some different choices to work with. He may just walk away to avoid his thoughts. But he might react in kind even though that 'kind' has taken on a very different character. The conflict could end abruptly as if it never was. Sometimes some amazing things happen when one person refuses to play this game. When you have nothing left within you that someone else's negativity can connect with, you've got it made. You become aware that you have the mighty power within to handle any situation.

Of course, there is a word of caution for anyone trying this for the first time. We need to be very careful that the feeling we are sending out is real. In other words, that genuine Love is coming from your heart - that you are not doing this from a position of superiority because that will come through and undo your good work for sure. It has to be real and genuine. So in that scenario, who has the power? When you are connected to your real power, anyone who would have conflict with you hasn't got a prayer, if you will pardon the expression.

There is indeed a better way. And it can be done without compromising ourselves in the least. But I don't want any misunderstanding. We are not talking about belittling ourselves in any way. It's the other way around.

It might take a little doing to see the wisdom of an acquiescent approach, but there is a larger picture coming through. When we see that, rather than belittling ourselves, we will be enlarging ourselves beyond anything we normally aspire to.

***

Mahatma means 'great soul'. We are all great souls, even if it doesn't seem like it sometimes. But every once in a while we get an example of a great soul to remind us of what we are really made of. Some person, who is the same as you and me except they worked at remembering their real nature, appears on the scene. Someone who worked, studied, and did whatever necessary to shed these false perceptions until they were successful, enabled them to know and became the truth.

Mahatma Gandhi came by the title 'Mahatma' because he earned it. He gave us an example of our greatness by demonstration - an example of our potential for all to see and be inspired by. He embodied the point we are trying to make here.

Mahatma Gandhi won the fight to liberate the people of India from colonial rule by non-resistance. Some of that action is even documented on film. The British soldiers lost their will to fight because there was nothing to fight against.

It's a lot like playing ping pong although the stakes are a little higher. With ping pong, two people are hitting a ball back and forth to each other. If one of the participants chooses not to participate and doesn't hit the ball back, the game ends. Now I know that war is a little more than a ping pong game and the emotions involved are considerably different and can't really be compared. The participants in a war have a little more to lose and have a monumental barrier in front of them in terms of letting go and transforming the emotions involved.

But Gandhi had that covered. He didn't let it get started. He instructed his soldiers not to respond and certainly not to initiate any aggression. His defense was no defense. It was called passive resistance and it worked. What an astounding achievement to hold to that ideal in the most trying circumstance. But his much greater accomplishment was to instill that belief and discipline in the people he was leading. Mahatma Gandhi demonstrated the true meaning of the word meek and redefined it for us. To be meek means to be in your true power. And look at the results. They got their country back. How's that for inheriting the earth?

We can move into the new world to which we aspire with relative ease. The big and important difference for us, as previously mentioned, is that we no longer have to go through the rigours and deprivation of an austere lifestyle to get connected. And we certainly are not expected to be martyrs. The time we are in is especially made to facilitate reconnection - reconnection with ease and simplicity. And part of that facilitation, besides the fact that God has been cranking up the volume, is the opportunity to take advantage of past accomplishments by using them as examples of what works.

These battles of history – or non-battle as in the case of Gandhi - represent the conflict within ourselves that we can take on if we want to be part of changing the world. That personal inner battle may not seem to be anywhere near as glorious as what the great ones performed, but it actually is. Each and every individual inner conflict won is glorious - a great victory because it is the only one that each of us has complete jurisdiction over. It is also glorious and a great victory because it's the same battles that all the great ones fought and won: *'for so persecuted they the prophets which were before you'*. And our battle is glorious for another reason: It takes courage to take on the only real enemy, that enemy represented by all the error and misunderstanding that we have adopted.

That truly is the final battle after which there can never be conflict on earth ever again. This last battle is fought in solitude, without fanfare or notice from the outer world. Each of us has only to take that little bit of initiative to point ourselves in the right direction. It won't happen by itself. It can't because of our free will - our complete autonomy. We must freely choose to seek truth and release the obstructions that block the light. It starts with each of us. The final war takes place where all wars started: Within each of us as individuals. That's World War 3 and it involves everybody.

Give to him that asketh thee,
and from him that would borrow of thee turn not thou away.

It comes down to giving. The concept of giving as part of our nature follows the recognition of agreement as part of our nature. And here it is, where it will do the most good and where our greatest challenge is. What better place to learn about giving than with someone who is making unreasonable demands of us. It might not be the best place to start getting the concept, but it is the best place to understand the true meaning of giving. If we can remember our real nature in a challenging situation like this, we've got it. Our greatest challenge is also our greatest opportunity for advancement.

Chapter Seven

LOVE

*Ye have heard that it hath been said,
Thou shalt love thy neighbour, and hate thine enemy.
But I say unto you,
Love your enemies,
bless them that curse you,
do good to them that hate you,
and pray for them which despitefully use you, and persecute you;
That ye may be the children of your Father which is in heaven:
for he maketh his sun to rise on the evil and on the good,
and sendeth rain on the just and on the unjust.
For if ye love them which love you,
what reward have ye?
do not even the publicans the same?
And if ye salute your brethren only,
what do ye more than others?
do not even the publicans so?*

A silly mathematical riddle floated around my high school for a while: Three men rented a hotel room together. It was the last room available and the clerk charged them 30 dollars. Later, the clerk reconsidered because the price was a little high – yeah, I'm that old. So, he sent the bellboy up with 5 dollars as a refund. But rather than try to divide 5 by 3, the bellboy decided to keep 2 dollars and give each of the men 1 dollar. Now, that means each man only paid 9 dollars. So do the math, as they say: 3 times 9 is 27 and the bellboy kept 2 which makes 29. But the original amount was 30. Where did the other dollar go? As I said, that was a long time ago and we took that question seriously and even managed to get one of our teachers confused with it.

It's not hard to see that this bit about loving your enemy is an update. There is quite a gap between the two. Let's see if we can see how the new includes the old and expand on it. How does loving your enemy fulfill the old law of hating your enemy?

That was a trick question. I just wanted to see if you were paying attention. We often do not get the answers we need because we ask the wrong questions. And we ask the wrong questions because we ask questions from outside the boundaries of truth. We ask questions about the darkness because we live in darkness. But it would make more sense to ask questions about the light because we live in darkness. The above question was an example of a question asked from darkness about darkness.

We are not going from hating our enemy to loving our enemy. We are going from loving our neighbour to loving our enemy - from Love to an expansion of Love and from Love to greater Love. That trick question was more than a trick. It was dishonest and misleading. A better question on the subject would be: How does loving your enemy fulfill the law of loving your neighbour? That's the real question and one that is answerable. That's the kind of question asked from one in the darkness who is inquiring about the light - big difference.

Now the answer is obvious and very simple. There is a smooth transition like everything else we have updated. The answer to my deliberately misleading question is this: We had to start somewhere with Love, so we do the easy things first. Loving your neighbour was a good place to start and it still is. Even now, what chance do we have of loving an enemy unless we have had at least some practice at loving someone a little easier to Love? From a first getting a concept of Love, we can take it further. We can go all the way with Love and take our experience of it - the final step. We are ready to understand Love and understand ourselves. Love understood completely and put into practice puts us back in touch with our true nature. This makes use of the old and fulfills, just like all the other updates did.

But to get back to this thing about asking the right question: An honest question contains its answer within. Expanding our Love to our enemies after learning to Love those near to us is contained in the question about fulfilling the law of loving your neighbour. It is an honest question about light, asking how to get to more light. But asking how one could be capable of loving an enemy from a position of hate is a lot like the question about the vanishing dollar. The honest calculation renders the question invalid: 3 times 9 is 27, minus the 2 that the bellboy kept makes 25, which is the real number we need to balance since it is the new total after 5 was subtracted from 30. Adding instead of subtracting was the misleading part.

The problem with living in the darkness is the expectation of continued darkness. We ask questions designed to perpetuate the darkness. So we have to raise our expectations considerably for all that we are learning, but especially for this one:

LOVE.

This next step is about Love. Actually, every step is about Love, but this is Love defined. Therefore, it is us defined. This tells us who we are in the plainest possible language. When we start to remember the true meaning of Love and the truth about ourselves, we see everything from a different perspective.

It's not that hard. All that is required in getting back to what we are, as previously mentioned, is just releasing everything that is unlike what we are. Let me tell you a little story of how that happened to me way back a generation or two ago. Way back when I didn't know what I was doing, but it worked. There is nothing like innocence to facilitate success. I think that's where beginner's luck comes from - Innocence. I have yet to surpass what I accomplished when I first became aware of another way of doing things.

When this story took place, and unlike most of my life alone and backing up big rigs, my work involved other people. One person, in particular, played a key role in my activities. We needed to work together cooperatively to be successful. Unfortunately, the person in question seemed not to have any concept of cooperation. Or at least he had not given me any reason to believe that he had any understanding of what his job entailed.

Now, for some strange reason, I have always taken work seriously and insisted on accomplishment one way or another. And aside from that, I was also an extremely intolerant young fellow in those days. So we had a serious conflict - a daily ritual of unpleasant exchanges. Well, not so much exchanges as a barrage of insults and sarcasm directed to my co-worker from me. He seldom engaged or responded to my insults but rather, now that I look back, I believe he was silently attending to finding ways to be even less cooperative. We had a hopeless deadlock. Things were not going well. I was so very irritated in my work life that I was considering making a change. I considered quitting.

But fate intervened. I became ill. I got the flu and missed a week of work, at the end of which time I was still ill. Although I hadn't fully recuperated, I went back to work because I thought it was time - not very smart. I promptly got a worse case of the flu and then learned that it had turned into pneumonia. I say found out because I was living alone at the time and wasn't well enough to get to a doctor. But I knew I had a bad problem. I felt dreadful and could barely manage to get myself out of bed to get a little sustenance from time to time. It's one thing to be seriously ill and it's one thing to be alone, but the two together is not something that anyone would plan. But I had learned one thing at least. This time, I allowed myself plenty of time to recuperate.

Just previous to this, I had stumbled onto a book that was not in my normal range of reading. But it did get my attention and it was the beginning of my interest in the topic at hand. The book was quite esoteric and made reference to God which I didn't have any interest in, but most of the book was fascinating and gave me an entirely new perspective. O.K. we're finally getting to the crunch here. I reread this book several times during my recuperation, and I don't know for sure if it was the particular state I was in from having battled a serious illness while alone or what it was, but I do know I was in a far more receptive state than was my normal. At any rate, I took the content of the book to heart.

Part of the book had especially caught my attention - being accepting of others. It was suggested that complete acceptance of others will, and must, have a dramatic impact on our everyday interactions. Of course, acceptance of any kind - let alone total acceptance - was quite the opposite of my normal stance at the time. But as mentioned, a combination of circumstances had caused me to entertain this different point of view.

When I finally went back to work, I was keenly looking forward to trying out my newfound 'wisdom'. And of course, the first thing I did was to employ my new strategy to affect harmony with my antagonist. But it didn't work! Now what? I was shocked. I was totally convinced of the validity of my new findings and outlook. Nothing changed. My co-worker was as uncooperative and remiss in his duties as ever. But I just couldn't leave this alone. Rather, 'it' wouldn't leave me alone. It kept running through my mind. So during that process, it came to me to playback and examine all of the activities that had been in my mind while I had been practicing my newfound philosophy. With close examination, I began to realize that I had been running another program at the same time. Yes, I had been accepting, but now with this careful re-examination, I was remembering thinking at the same time, that this person truly is a dodo.

That's not TOTAL acceptance Albert! Try again! The next day I decided to pull out all the stops. I would be totally and unconditionally accepting no matter what - even if it made me look bad because I didn't get my work done. That was the hard part. To be prepared to allow myself to look bad by not getting my work done was a big hurdle. Something I would never do. I was a real fanatic about getting my work done. I would never allow myself to be caught out like that. But I said the hell with it and decided to go for broke.

Are you ready for this? The change in that man is something I marvel at to this day. He just couldn't do enough for me. He immediately and ever after became cooperation personified. My work became easy and a pleasure. We even got to like one another. We didn't become friends to the point of association outside of work, but we did develop a fondness and respect for each other.

So what did I really do way back then when I didn't know what I was doing? What did I do that was so effective? I said it was beginner's luck, but that's all I needed. That's all you need. I succeeded because I didn't know any better. All I did is get out of my own way. Love happens all by itself when there is nothing in the way obstructing it. There is a constant flow of Love always available, ready for action. It is Love that does the work and cuts through all complications.

It's a little humbling to realize that I did nothing at all. In fact, it is for the very reason that I did nothing, that something good was caused to happen, which means that good was always ready to come about, just waiting for me to get out of the way. It was my constant barrage of animosity and less than complimentary comments towards my co-worker that had been causing the problem.

Therefore, problems do not exist in our natural state. Problems have to be caused, created. We have to go to a lot of trouble to create problems. Think how much easier the alternative is. And isn't that quite an understatement? Easier? No kidding! How much easier is it to just let the natural harmony of the universe take place rather than work hard at making up ways to make things difficult?

Love is like water behind the tap. It's always ready to flow as soon as the tap is opened. The tap in the kitchen is what is stopping the water from running into the sink. As soon as you open the tap, the water runs. It was always there and under pressure, but you don't notice it until you let it run. But you trust that it will be there. Of course the city utilities commission or whatever it is that supplies your water is fallible and it could happen that something went wrong and the water stopped. Not so with Love. Love never fails. It's been put at the ready forever. If for some reason it doesn't seem to work, there has to be a restriction of some sort. Love can't fail and total acceptance opens the tap. It's that simple. And the tap is either open or it is not. Even a little restriction stops the tap from opening at all. It's like the computer that doesn't do what I want for some reason. That reason is usually me. The chances are that I have forgotten one little thing or there is something I don't know about or I've just plain made an error.

My computer is fallible so I may have done everything right without getting results. But I always know where to look when something doesn't work in my personal world. The only possible impediment to the Divine is me.

As we practice opening the tap, we get better at it. We eventually get so good at it that we are capable of opening the tap even in the most trying situations. And then finally the day comes when we see no reason to ever close the tap. So we practice keeping it open all the time. And when that practice is perfected we forever after express our real selves, which is Love, at all times. Simple? Of course it is. Nobody ever said getting connected to spirit was complicated. If you want something complicated, just start looking at all the barriers to Love we have created since I don't know when. Was that useful? Well as I have said before, it kept us in the dark for a very long time and we must have done it for a reason. But time's up.

That's what all the changes in the world are about. The incoming wave of truth is bringing out all the old falseness so that we can see it, let it go, and express our true selves. And that is the real challenge for all of us, collectively and individually. The tap is not hard to open. It's the determination to do so despite a vested interest in hanging onto the emotions of the past. It's only by letting our past dictate our actions that we complicate things and delay our success. But we have covered this before in several different ways and I even warned that I would cover it again. Still, there it is. The answer is always Love and the blockages are always everything we have created that didn't have Love in the recipe.

Loving those near and dear to us - the ones who Love us back - is easy, but it doesn't stretch us beyond our normal boundaries. It doesn't challenge us to our purpose or to finding out what we are really made of. We can do better. A lot better. It's in our very nature to do so - that nature that comes out when we Love. So we are to Love indiscriminately as God does. That's how we will experience what we have forgotten about ourselves. That we are as God.

But that doesn't mean that I can say that I know what Divine Love is. And I certainly cannot say that I am a personification thereof at this point. I've had moments of something like Love on a personal level and I've had glimpses of what we are seeking, but I have never been able to truly define or completely understand Divine Love. But those glimpses have been enough to keep me going no matter what. Once you get just a little taste of the real thing, the world as we know it loses its appeal.

It is understandable and to be expected that we don't really know or are able to feel what Divine Love is. That's the very thing we are separated from. So it is the acknowledgment of that simple fact that can get us started back towards it. We cannot know what real Love is in the state we are in. If we really knew Divine Love, we wouldn't be doing all this. Getting connected to Love in its truest sense defines our whole challenge. Everything else we are learning about leads up to that - leads us to the Love that we are and have forgotten. So how do we get back to it? How do we feel that which we seem to have lost the feel for? How do we actually summon Divine Love when we can't be sure what it feels like anymore? How do we get started on it?

We need a bridge - a method of bridging that gap. And that's why I recommend total acceptance. Total acceptance allows Divine Love to flow even though we may not yet be aware of, or be able to *feel* that Love. That's the bridge. And the practice of total acceptance is the process of crossing that bridge over and over again until we see and feel and know something different.

Practicing total acceptance until it is an automatic process can take us safely home. Using that bridge can be our defining activity. Then Love flows through and we, therefore, begin to experience and know the Love that we are. Then Divine Love is gradually understood and known because it is *felt*. And then we become aware that God is Love. Not just as a concept, but as real knowing. And more, that knowing that we are created from and of Love becomes an actual *feeling* of knowing. We become aware of our true nature again. We remember.

Love is the cause of creation. Creation cannot take place without Love. Therefore, we cannot create anything constructive without Love. Love permeates all of creation. So to get in on the act, we need to get back to our true nature.

We have only to be the Love that we are. We do not have to recreate ourselves. We have only to remove all that is artificial and by which we have redefined ourselves. We have only to remove all that is obstructing our real nature to get back to our real nature.

But that trip back is usually a process. We went through a process of getting away from ourselves. It was done little by little. It sort of snuck up on us or we could never have tolerated it. We got used to expressing a little less of our real nature and then got used to a little less than that from that new level and so on and so on for generations, to get this low. We went through a process of removing ourselves from what we are by imagining all kinds of things that we are not. And we let that become a habit until we truly redefined ourselves. We have redefined ourselves in terms so vastly different from what we really are that it is almost impossible to find common ground for comparison. This means that we have a lot of information, beliefs and complicated ways of being that are blocking Love from coming through.

So back to the bridge:

That bridge can take us across with ease. That's not the problem. Our bridge takes us across the flow of all that impedes Love. But we don't want to forget about the stream or the quality of that stream for which the bridge was built. That stream is polluted. Our metaphorical stream is filled with anything and everything we have ever done, thought about, or have otherwise been involved in. Our incredible subconscious minds faithfully record all. That stream we want to cross is our stream of consciousness as it is now. And it is what we want to get beyond and leave behind forever. But using a bridge to avoid swimming or otherwise crossing a stream does not eliminate the stream. The purpose of the bridge is to get to the other side and visit reality so that we have something to go by - so that we can obtain the needed strength and understanding to be able to see the stream for what it really is and do something about it. Once we start to see the reality on the other side of the bridge, we quite naturally see the stream as it is - filled with the pollution adopted from our fictitious world. Our glimpse of the Truth has given us the strength and motivation to deal with the stream. Our course of action becomes crystal clear. We want to stop all pollution from entering the stream and we want to clean it up. Once we are introduced to the clear waters of Truth again, dissolving all that pollutes becomes an all-consuming passion.

How do I know this? Because I did it the hard way. I took an unnecessary 30-year detour wallowing in the murky waters of the past. A word of caution: My success with my co-worker way back then was the beginning, not the end of learning. That's why I recommend continual use of the bridge while clearing the stream. In the meantime, we cannot swim in it, drink from it, bathe in it, or make use of it in any way. But you can't ignore it either. Yes, it has to be cleaned up, but we can't do that from within the stream. And that's the tricky part and the part that requires focus. That stream will become more noticeable every time we cross the bridge for two reasons. Each trip to the other side will bring about a stronger sense of Truth and therefore renders the stream to be in even sharper contrast. And two, the stream is very demanding of your attention because that's where the habit of attention is. As we adopt new habits, the old ones become more demanding.

Time out.

The above reference to a bridge and a stream of course is a metaphor. It is my preferred means of working towards understanding spirit. I wonder if any real learning begins without it. We need the metaphor because we have nothing with which to refer when trying to add to our learning when it comes to matters of the spirit. But I will explain the above in plain language as well. My purpose is to be explicit. The main purpose of this whole endeavour is to make sure that we don't leave anyone behind. I know there are some of you brave souls who explored the darkness to such an extent as to become almost completely lost in it. You have done something that I do not have the capacity to consider, let alone do. I did not realize until later in life that many people are so totally ensconced in this world as to believe in it completely. It never occurred to me to take life seriously. What I mean is - I also went through a long time of knowing nothing else but this physical world, but I never saw life the way some people seem to. I got lost too, but I knew I was lost, that's the difference. I became confused and dysfunctional by this world, but it always seemed like a play to me and I just assumed that everyone else felt the same. But I have come to realize that that has been an error on my part. A lot of people seem to take life seriously.

So, my desire to be explicit stems from an enormous respect for anyone who has worked on project earth with such devotion as to abandon the lifeline to home completely. I feel compelled to explain things like our bridge and the polluted stream in plain language for all the courageous people who have gone beyond the expected boundaries with this little game of pretending - this game of pretending to be so much less than we really are.

O.K., we're back and the following is the explicit explanation of total acceptance, minus the metaphor:

Total acceptance is a very powerful method of getting us back to our real nature, so powerful that it is worthy of a little respect and at least an equal amount of caution. It is so powerful that it cannot fail. If it seems to fail, we have only to go back and find what residue is left within total acceptance that renders it not actually total. And then try again. You will know when success comes. You might not notice it with those that are easy to accept, but you will notice it with anyone or anything that you have had difficulty accepting - as in *love your enemy*. There will be a dramatic change that leaves no doubt. It will leave no doubt because you will be looking at the results of Divine Love in action and you will see something tangibly different.

But even though that change is indeed a dramatic change for the better, it will present a challenge that can be overlooked. And if that challenge is overlooked, it will defeat the purpose of total acceptance.

Here is that challenge, why it can be overlooked, how it can be overlooked, and what happens when it is: That dramatic change I am referring to can be a very giddy experience. Such success is usually quite exhilarating. It can leave you feeling that you have arrived - that you can handle anything. And there is some truth in that. It is the power of Divine Love you have tapped into and activated and Divine Love can handle anything. But that same great power of Divine Love brings out and highlights all that is not of Love. How can it not? When Love enters the equation, all else becomes obvious by contrast. Therefore, you will become much more aware of all that is less than desirable. And that's the pitfall. That immediate sense of an ability to handle anything can be misleading.

Yes, Divine Love can handle anything, but our little exercise in total acceptance was only a beginning. It does not mean that we can handle anything at this early stage and it most certainly does not, and cannot mean that we have that power and ability as our own. This is why the great ones put so much emphasis on humility. A humble approach to spirit, Truth, Love, God, is the ability to recognize that the power you are working with is not that of the person you believe yourself to be – not in this present state.

I know that this humble thing can be a bit of a stopper, but only because there has been too much misunderstanding for too long about humility. To be humble is not to put yourself down. It is to raise yourself up! It means accepting yourself where you are so that you can go from there. That's all being humble means. It means acknowledging that things are not what they could be, that we are not connected to our real selves. This takes us back to square one - being open to something better.

Blessed are the poor in spirit: for theirs is the kingdom of heaven

And we can throw in the next two Beatitudes while we're at it. The three together form a base and make up what we need to get started. We need to acknowledge that we come from a sense of powerlessness. Even people who are very successful in the world have an underlying sense of powerlessness that stems from being separated from Source, whether or not there is an awareness of this.

So for anyone who has chosen to use our bridge:

Your total acceptance allowed Love to do its work, but that's all you accomplished so far. Yes, that's a great accomplishment, but, as mentioned, it can be misleading. It is so easy at this point to overlook the fact that you have done nothing yourself. Even though you just had a huge success by employing the power of Divine Love, that power has not yet been established as a *permanent* part of your consciousness. As we all know, establishing Divine Love within ourselves is a process. And during that process, we are vulnerable to all else because all else is still predominant within. So, it is important that the kind of success we are referring to here is understood and seen in proper perspective. Otherwise, it can quite easily be too distracting and we defeat our purpose. It's easy to overlook or forget or otherwise ignore real cause at this point - to not give credit where credit is due. Spirit is very subtle and has no way of informing you that it is the power behind your accomplishment.

If we want to use total acceptance as a method of getting back to our real identity, we have to understand what's really happening. Otherwise, we just get ourselves in nothing but trouble. The main hazard with what we are doing here is that it works so well. And the subtle trap is the inclination to accept what was accomplished as our own doing. That stops the process dead in its tracks! As soon as you say, 'I did this', the process automatically stops. Love was activated because you got out of your own way. 'I did this', is getting back in your own way and shutting the door to the flow of spirit. We are better off without our method than to use it without understanding, without an understanding of what is actually taking place.

Complete understanding of what we are doing here starts with acknowledging the source of the power we are activating - that power we became separated from and are trying to get back to. Understanding and using total acceptance means the full realization that it is a *method* of getting reconnected. It is not reconnection itself. It is meant to be used to handle all things that give trouble until all things that give trouble no longer exist. And when all things that give trouble no longer exist, you will know yourself differently. You will know that you have become the Love that you are. You will know that you are pure Divine Love because there will no longer be anything other than Love capable of getting your attention. Even the seeming disparities of the world will be seen with and in Love. And at that point, total acceptance is not something you will consider because total acceptance is built into Love. Love is always totally accepting. Love makes no demands.

Healing or otherwise dealing with all that is unlike Love cannot be done without Love. That's why I call total acceptance a bridge. It is meant to be used to *visit* our true selves while we are in the process of releasing anything that is unlike our true selves. Once that process is complete, you will no longer need the bridge because you will have become the bridge. And you will know that you have become the bridge because the polluted stream will no longer exist. (Sorry about that; I just had to revert to the metaphor.)

So stay on the bridge no matter what - even if it's slippery and it demands all of your attention. It's worth it. I know because I took a great detour. I did not stay focused on the bridge long enough to have it established as part of myself. The process of bringing up all else, not to mention a major pattern of self-deprecation, overwhelmed me. I had a lot of stuff. A little less stuff and a little more sanity would have made it easier I'm sure. But a lot more perseverance would definitely have been the answer.

One more thing about how to access Divine Love: There is one thing more important than all of the above put together: Self Love. The ability to Love oneself is the greatest shortcut of all. Anyone who can truly Love herself or himself doesn't need a road to Love because they already have it established. When you can truly Love yourself, loving others is automatic. But I am coming from the assumption that the vast majority of us have a lot of trouble with self Love. That's why our method is necessary. With total acceptance, Love for oneself is involved incidentally. We gain Love for ourselves without even knowing it. The act of totally accepting others is a loving act to yourself because at that moment there is nothing unlike Love flowing through you. It's the best way to self Love because you don't realize that you're doing it and you, therefore, do not give yourself an opportunity to cancel it. Some of us have such a strong inability to Love ourselves that we sabotage our efforts at every opportunity. So we usually come to Love ourselves by practicing loving others. Self Love sort of sneaks up on you without you realizing what has happened.

And there is a way to crank this whole thing up to the highest level and get it all done with, forever: Loving those most difficult to Love is the most powerful thing to do.

But I say unto you, Love your enemies,
bless them that curse you, do good to them that hate you,
and pray for them which despitefully use you, and
persecute you.

The greater the negativity directed towards you, the greater the requirement to put out the positive, and the greater is the benefit. The benefit increases because of the greater power that was activated.

And the result of loving your enemy:

That ye may be the children of your Father
which is in heaven.

The act of loving your enemies activates the memory of your true identity. Love the person or persons who are the hardest to Love. That will get you there quicker than anything. That's why He said Love your enemy. So that we can see what it's like to express our true selves. It takes you back to and reminds you of your unchangeable nature. It reminds you that you *are* Love and that Love is your job description.

for he maketh his sun to rise on the evil and on the good,
and sendeth rain on the just and on the unjust.

That's the way God gets things done. With no thought of anything but Love. Love is lavished on everyone and everything at all times and without any opposing force because Love is all there is. There is no opposing force other than our misunderstanding.

So what all this means is that making that big turnaround is how we get hooked into our real power. We don't make much progress toward our return to truth and reality by only loving those that Love us. That just more or less maintains things as they are.

For if ye love them which love you,
what reward have ye?
do not even the publicans the same?

*And if ye salute your brethren only,
what do ye more than others?
do not even the publicans so?*

  But lest there be misunderstanding, be it known that loving our enemies does not ever imply any kind of agreement in any way with anything negative. It does not mean that we could possibly consider condoning misdeeds of any kind. When we love our enemies, we are not loving unacceptable behaviour. We are loving the person separate from the behaviour. We are directing attention to the perfection that exists beyond the behaviour. That's what total acceptance means and does. And that's why it works so well. It addresses the eternal truth about a person rather than the particular behaviour of the moment. It's a silent reminder of reality, to both of you. When you address anyone on that level, you are opening the tap to allow the participation of the cause of all things. Once you bring some Truth into the mix, everything changes because anything that is not of Truth has no power of its own. Anything not of Truth collapses as soon as that which had been sustaining it is removed. Fear and hatred are artificial and must have a constant supply of negative energy to sustain them. The only way anyone can continue hatred toward us is by us helping him out with it.
  But we are saying remove that help so that the supply of fuel for negative behaviour is shut off. Love doesn't have a fuel supply problem, because Love is in infinite supply. Love is the constant of the universe. Not fear or hatred or anything else false that we have created during our time of separation. Our enemies are not the people with whom we have difficulty. Our real enemy is misunderstanding, lack of awareness, and any and all misconception/fear that we have picked up along the way.
  Love is the essence and the fuel of the universe. Therefore loving or not loving is just not a consideration in

terms of creation. Love is how creation comes about. It is how we, the earth, and all else were created. As apprentice Gods, or children of God, as we are referred to in biblical terms, we are learning how God does things so that we can do the same. That's what we are all about. And that's why we have this detailed reminder of what we are and what we came here to do.

THEREFORE

*Be ye therefore perfect,
even as your Father which is in heaven is perfect.*

I have an older brother who is a genius. He was a truck driver for part of his working life, but that's about the only thing we have in common. But he didn't just drive. He always found a way to use his many talents no matter what he did. Hauling hay is an example. He developed a unique way of building a load so that it was secure. But that wasn't good enough for him. It also had to have an aesthetic appearance. I don't think he ever fully appreciated his talents. To him all this was normal.

But where he truly displayed his brilliance, at least with the part of him that is a trucker, was in hauling cattle. He had that down to a fine art. Driving with a load of livestock is not that big of a deal except that it is important to drive smoothly, especially at the beginning to get the cattle used to the movement. But loading and unloading are where the real talent comes in. I'm sure everything else was secondary to him, even though we never discussed it.

The cattle are usually in corrals so it's just a matter of backing the trailer up to a chute, opening one or more gates, and then chasing the cattle out and up the ramp to the trailer. Unloading is a similar procedure. That's the normal way it is done, and other than my brother, I have never known anybody to do it any different.

Here's the scenario: My brother comes into the stockyards with a semi-trailer loaded with cattle. He backs up to the chute. As usual, there are some people around to receive the load and to see that the cattle go to the proper holding area. And as always, these people come to help because it usually takes several people to prod the cattle to move. But my dear brother has a different request for these would-be helpers. He informs them in his commanding way, that if they really want to help, they are to quietly leave the area and remain silent some distance away.

He then goes into action. Everything is in readiness - the open tailgate and his green coveralls. He calmly and gently positions himself near the cattle with his back to them. He hunches over – way over. He pulls the top of his coveralls over his head. Slowly, he begins walking down the chute. And after a little time, one of his passengers takes notice and begins walking in my brother's direction. Once this process starts, it quickly escalates. One after another, the cows follow the crowd – who are following my brother. Soon, there are no cattle in the trailer. Only then is his human audience allowed to venture near.

I didn't get it. He had to explain it to me. I don't mind. I have been aware of his talents ever since I can remember. The green coveralls? So simple it's laughable. The grass that the cows eat is green. They look favourably to the colour green. Cows could be colour blind for all I know but I'm sure that there is something about green that gives them the green light. And the hunched over? Well, he just wants the cows to be unaware that there is any human involvement. And above all - the quiet. Then it's like nature - the way things are in the pasture. And lastly, the cows are hungry if they have traveled any distance, so a little green is quite welcome I'm sure. All a very natural process. No fuss - the usual commotions don't ensue as it does when forcibly unloading cattle. Just a simple operation that only requires the human element at its best.

Divine harmony always works with simplicity. And genius is the simple act of being tuned in. The most beautiful accomplishments always come about with minimal effort. If you could see what is involved in the normal operation of loading or unloading cattle and then compare that to what I have described above, you would have a glimpse of Divine Harmony. A little preview of perfection.

To aspire to perfection might seem beyond reach while we are surrounded by imperfection, but perfection is our natural state. Therefore there is only one worthy activity in life - to continually acknowledge and release anything that is not of Divine harmony within us, in whatever way we can. And once we get going on that little project, life starts to make sense. It is only then that we can truly begin to understand the meaning of life. This is why the question of meaning has always plagued us. Most of us feel too far off track to fully address that question in our present state. But be assured we will address it before we are done here.

In the meantime, this is a major therefore. This is the therefore for everything we have covered so far. It is the natural conclusion from the content of the opening statements. And it is the conclusion from each and all of the updates combined. And it is the natural conclusion from what we might expect from a final update.

And it is more. It also conclusively defines us. This is where all this has been going right from the beginning. We've covered everything about who we are and what our potential is. And we've covered how to start fulfilling that potential by focusing on the qualities that would lead us back to truth. With the constant reminder that we are like God, we have been redefining ourselves, culminating with the reminder of our true nature as Love.

The clear inference all along with the reference to us as children of God and that we have the ability to overcome every kind of adversity, not to mention the radical quality of meekness, has been preparing us for this moment - preparing us for the full realization that we are created in God's image and that we are perfect beings with the capacity to express perfection. That's where this has been taking us and where it will continue to take us. That's the purpose of our endeavour here - to get back to knowing ourselves and regain the ability to express that knowing.

We have the ability and the potential, and indeed, it is our destiny to manifest perfection. Perfection already exists. Everything already is. Infinity is the substance just waiting for conscious direction. Love requires no force to do its work, and infinity doesn't have a supply problem. Perfection comes about with absolute ease and simplicity, and with the least possible effort. We express our perfection by allowing, *by w*orking with nature by deploying our real nature.

So I hope this forever removes any doubt about whether or not this is the final update. Unless someone can tell me how to improve on perfection, I'm not expecting any further updates.

No, we're probably not going to improve on perfection, but we do need to look at what is in the way of it. As things stand at the time of this writing, there are still a number of barriers within us that stand in the way of the expression of our perfection. And we just happen to have some of that pointed out to us in the next section.

Chapter Eight

SECRECY

*Take heed that ye do not your alms before men,
to be seen of them:
otherwise ye have no reward of your Father
which is in heaven.
Therefore when thou doest thine alms,
do not sound a trumpet before thee,
as the hypocrites do in the synagogues and in the streets,
that they may have glory of men.
Verily I say onto you,
They have their reward.
But when thou doest alms,
let not thy left hand know what thy right hand doeth:
That thine alms may be in secret:
and thy Father which seeth in secret himself
shall reward thee openly.*

I heard a story about how time was kept in a small town. It was done in a rather strange way. The man who operated the local radio station walked to work every day and his route took him by the watch repair shop. He always carefully noted the time displayed on a big clock in the window so that he could be sure to announce the time accurately. This was a daily ritual he had practiced for years. But one day he had a bit of extra time and stopped to talk to the man at the clock shop. He asked the repairman where he got the right time. The repairman replied, "I listen to your radio, I get it from you."

If our faithful timekeeper/radio announcer was off just a few seconds a day, it is conceivable that over a period of years, the time could be so far off that the people might wonder why it was getting dark at noon.

Now let's imagine that our small town is completely isolated and that the radioman, having realized his mistake, decides to take full responsibility for announcing the right time. He might remember that the sun sets at a particular time on the longest day of the year and go from there. He could even use other markers from the sun for periodic checks and be assured that he was reasonably close - certainly a lot closer than by the previous method.

We measure time by how long it takes the earth to revolve on its axis and by how long it takes the earth to complete an orbit around the sun. We can go beyond that if we want because the sun is not stationary. But for practical purposes, we use the sun as the centre and the constant. That works rather well. We have night and day and we have the seasons. It's all very predictable. Although, in more primitive times, certain people had very important ceremonies to call back the sun. They believed that the sun was leaving and that it was up to them to do the appropriate things and to pray to make the sun come back.

We are quite enlightened now as far as understanding what causes the seasons and we never worry about it. We take it all for granted. That's just the way it is. It's all very reliable. Spring will follow winter. It's so simple it's not worth mentioning. Yet we are living in primitive times when it comes to understanding the simplicity of our own nature.

For example, running around expecting validation from each other is about as enlightened as the clock man and the radioman using the information they got from each other to set the time. Expecting validation from each other is no more enlightened than calling back the sun each year. The days will get longer in the northern hemisphere after the winter solstice and we are perfect Divine beings. Those are givens. Nothing needs doing and no ceremonies are necessary to accomplish these things. I am not going to worry about how long the sun will exist and I am not going to worry about eternity or my part in it. The gift of what I am will not be rescinded. But we did get quite a long way off track by measuring ourselves by ourselves - by using each other as the standard.

We all want to be seen. We seem to need recognition, applause, or some kind of indication that we are worthy. One way or another, we demand that others do that for us. We have this need to be verified or validated. This compelling need is all subconscious of course, but why would that be? Why do we need others to inform us that we are OK? Why do we need the approval of others to feel good about ourselves? This need seems quite natural. Most of us do it to some degree or other. Some of us do it to an extreme and seem to need validation or notice of one kind or another, constantly. But is that really natural? Or is it only natural to our unnatural state?

Well then, if that's the case and those others who validate us also need validation, the obvious question is: Who is setting the standard?

We need something like the sun as a constant to measure ourselves by so that we don't mix up night and day. We have confused night with day and we've gotten so used to it that we no longer remember what the light is like.

The standard we are looking for is the light that is within us - the light that can only be found after we have removed all that obscures. Ability, talent, or capacity, is never our problem. We all have something unique to contribute to the world. Our real problem is finding a way to release all that restricts the expression of what we are. We suffer severe loss if we do not or will not remove the blocks that are in the way of our true self-expression. But that doesn't mean that most of us will be called on to do heroic things, except for one thing. To express your true self *is* heroic. Any person who is not expressing his or her true self cannot possibly be happy. The general dissatisfaction that most of us feel comes from our true self trying to get through.

But there is a greater loss involved than our happiness or fulfillment, within those of us who have not found a way to be ourselves: THE WORLD IS BEING SHORT-CHANGED AS WELL. Each of us is a vital piece of the puzzle in creating the picture of heaven on earth. The earth and heaven and God and the universe are all ready for this and only waiting for the rest of us to be ourselves too so that all the pieces fall into place and the puzzle will make sense and represent the picture on the box.

I don't mean this as criticism. Often the ones who are the most reticent are the ones who make the greatest contribution when the time is right. But we are being called as never before to make our individual contribution. Now is the time to get back in touch with that all-important forgotten part of ourselves. The time we are in lends itself to awakening to our real selves even as the necessity to do so increases by the crises in the world. We need all hands on deck to make this change. Once we are expressing who we are, each of us and all of us will be better off for it.

But how do we get there? And what stops most of us from stepping up to the plate? Most of us are reluctant to look at, if not unaware of our possibilities because we have paid too heavy a price to conform to the demands of the world. There is a big inhibiting factor here that needs to be brought out and given the light of day so that we can all see it for what it is. Once we see the truth about the untruth of our state of affairs, we will feel safe enough to give up whatever it is that is in the way of that true expression. And once we get a glimpse of the real truth about ourselves, we will have the courage to make whatever changes are necessary. Giving up that security blanket that seems so necessary in a false world will be done joyfully. That part within each and every one of us that we are trying to bring back to remembrance will come out to play.

So it's time to look at what makes us conform to that which is opposed to our real selves, which takes us back to the questions I posed about our need to be validated or noticed by others. What is it that compels us to look for validation from each other? It's something we exposed earlier. We continually seek validation because the validation we received as children wasn't real. What we received instead of validation was approval and recognition for conformity. We were consistently rewarded for conformity and disapproved of, or even ignored, for expressing what we really believed. The approval we received was relative to our conformity to the ways of the world. The pressure to conform was and is relentless and there wasn't much we could do but go along. But of course, we can't blame our parents or other adults for this because they went through the same process and are only passing on what they have learned to accept. That's how our fictitious world has been kept in perpetuity.

And as was also mentioned, when we are children, there is a point where we give in and accept the fact that we must pretend to be accepted. But that pretension means that we have effectively accepted an image of ourselves instead of what we really are. We function ever after with a counterfeit sense of self. We knew that then, and we know that now. We conformed to the lie, but deep down, we know better. Our real selves can never be completely subdued. So we are always expecting the truth about ourselves to be validated sometime, somehow, somewhere. The knowing of our real selves and the desire for the recognition of it by the world has stayed with us as a subconscious need.

That expectation is so strong that it permeates everything we do. Most of our actions incorporate that need automatically. That subconscious yearning finds ways of expression in the hope of having the truth about ourselves recognized. We did not get it from the people around us when we were children so we are still expecting it. That subconscious knowing of our basic goodness wants to be recognized but has no chance of success within the terms of this world. So what we are trying to do with our insatiable appetite for recognition is hear the truth about ourselves. We want someone to tell us what we never heard as children. Nothing will stop that powerful need for the confirmation of the truth about ourselves.

And we are right about the basic goodness of ourselves. But the problem comes from the fact that we have been taught to look to the outer world for answers. That subconscious knowing of our goodness is correct, but that knowing will not and cannot find the verification of its truth in this world of untruth. Our deep desire to have our real knowing about ourselves verified can only come out in a distorted way in this distorted world. Our desires and inclinations toward looking to the world for verification don't work. The world we have created in the absence of truth cannot possibly tell us the truth about ourselves.

So it might be a good idea to try something different. There is historical momentum behind the way the world functions, but that doesn't mean it can't be changed. The good news is that there has been a sharp increase in truth in all things lately. We are in an age where we demand truth and truth is readily forthcoming. The old ways are coming unraveled. This battle will be won. That's not the question. The only thing that is in question is whether or not we can do it easily. How many of us are going to find it difficult to let go of those old ways that are so ingrained?

So part of that difficulty is the issue at hand. We have an opponent worthy of a little respect here because a self-image is a key necessary component in the ability to function in the world as we know it. That's why it doesn't seem to make a lot of sense to redefine it, let alone give it up. As explained earlier, without a proper self-image we often become dysfunctional to some degree or other. We don't fit in; we don't become part of this world in any normal sense. Our self-image must be consistent with the general worldview if we are to function in a normal fashion.

And the only way we can function properly with the many details to attend to involved with this business of living is to put most things on autopilot. We learn to do things subconsciously or we couldn't possibly get through the day. Like walking for instance. That's a learned thing. Some people get so good at it that they can walk and chew gum at the same time. And maintaining an image of ourselves is an automatic thing too. It is something we had to learn and is ingrained into our consciousness. We have been taught this from an early age and most of us are extremely good at it. It is usually our number one priority and we learn it so well that we are capable of doing whatever it takes to maintain it. Even for those capable of walking and chewing gum at the same time, a continual and strong subconscious focus on the maintenance of a self-image is not diminished.

So let's go back to how this all starts, one more time: A newborn baby can't do any of what is suggested above and has a long way to go before starting on the basics. A new member of the world takes nearly two years just to get on topic for the more complicated issues like how we relate to one another. And even then, it takes a very important period of adjustment and learning to really get the hang of it. But most of these incredible little people get through that period. And low and behold, they get on with the business of relating more or less like everyone else.

But the biggest part of this adjustment, and the reason it is such a struggle for a little person, is this self-image thing. It's the part that is very difficult to accept. That's the sticker and the big hurdle even though it is your ticket for participation in this world. I must repeat - it is imperative that you create a belief about yourself that is consistent with the general belief system prevalent in the world if you want to get on that common ground within which to function. We are taught this from day one, and from every conceivable angle and source. Every person a child makes contact with automatically teaches that child the nature of the world by his very being and manner. Adults, older siblings, and or, anybody over the age of two, who have already made that adjustment, can't help but be that influence.

But it is important to realize that we pay an extremely high price for this conformity. A child pays the price of giving up the knowing inherent in his very being. Babies know! Take another look if you don't believe me. It's obvious a baby is in bliss. It's not because they know nothing. It's because they know everything! They are aware of God. But little by little, with the relentless influence of all the big people around them, they conform. They buy into the belief that you have to pretend to be something you are not. So we do indeed learn to pretend to be something we are not because the clear implication of the massive influence around us informs us that our natural belief about perfection is erroneous. And we become fearful like everyone else.

There is a terribly high price to pay for admission into this world. To give up the Truth about yourself as a perfect Divine child of God and replace it with a very limiting self-image imposed upon you is not a small thing. And worse, you can see the handwriting on the wall. Accepting this self-image of yourself will cause you to forget that truth about yourself. Who in his right mind would do this? Still, this is the admission fee and most people pay. But none of this process, and or, the conclusion drawn is done with the reasoning of an adult. The process of forced conformity by which we gradually lose our real and inherent knowing is all done subconsciously.

Most people successfully cross this big hurdle and become functional in this world complete with the necessary false image of self. And that's great except for one thing:

That necessary false image is unnecessary for where we are going now - for the change that's going on in the world. It's more than unnecessary. It gets in the way. And it is the big hurdle we are facing at this turning point of what we are trying to savvy right here and now. That's why it comes right after the conclusion that we are capable of displaying perfection. It is, quite naturally, the biggest stumbling block to reconnecting to spirit because that false self-image has become our *identity*. We believe that's what we are. How do you change what you are? Or why would you want to?

And even if you do want to change, the big stopper is that you have a subconscious memory of the original process - that process you went through of forgetting yourself and establishing that false sense of self. And that subconscious memory has to come through as a strong feeling against change. That was a harsh change and a change for the worse - much worse. It was a change in your very sense of identity from a Divine being to a very limited caricature of yourself as if you existed only as a physical being. So that memory, because it's subconscious, exists as an emotional residue on the conscious level - an emotional residue that consists of a very strong resistance to change. There is no way you're going through that again.

But we are indeed suggesting a similar change here. We're saying forget that self-image that you created and which cost you everything you had. Do away with your feeling of how you look in front of other people. Forget the importance of appearance, of how others perceive you - of being seen to be a good person; of being seen to be generous, kind, and all the other trappings necessary to maintain that image that you can't get along without in this world. Forget all that and spend your time instead practicing what we are learning here. And do it all so secretively that there is no chance whatsoever of being noticed. In other words, expect nothing from this world in terms of self-validation.

Take heed that ye do not your alms before men, to be seen of them otherwise ye have no reward of your Father which is in heaven.

Well, you can be sure any such endeavour is going to get opposition from a very different subconscious desire. May I repeat - you have a subconscious memory of going through this kind of a change before and it's not a good memory. There are very strong feelings of immense loss surrounding it. So here's the catch: Those strong feelings will be triggered as soon as you even consider making the kind of change advocated here. That's a very powerful psychological block worthy of respect. There has to be enormous resistance involved here. That resistance is built right into who we have come to believe ourselves to be. The resistance is so strong that most people don't even get on topic.

So we have to sneak up on our worthy opponent and work on it from more than one front. For starters, let's refrain from getting into the trap of looking at this and imagining that we can make this kind of shift all at once. We went through a long process to get so far removed from our Truth. So it is reasonable to assume that backtracking and reversing the process could challenge us just a bit. So I want to dig a little deeper into this problem to make sure we have everything we need to understand it. There could be a little more to this self-image problem than we might suspect.

The real problem is with the whole concept that a self-image is required at all. Why did we do this? That's the question we need to pose. And the simple answer is that the purpose of a self-created, self-image is to relate with one another. We all need to interact with one another within terms that we can understand in the world as it exists in the present state. Granted the world as we know it functions in fiction, but how else can we function in a fictitious world other than going along with the fiction?

So yes, we have a bit of challenge on our hands. But this whole self-image thing has a fatal flaw. We do have a secret weapon we can use. That secret weapon is the simple fact that the falseness we portray is not openly acknowledged. We do not talk about the self-image we have created for the very reason that it is false. We pretend that the self we show the world is real, but we know that it is not and so does everybody else. That's why it's impossible to feel fulfilled no matter how much attention we get. We are always looking for approval from others one way or another and we can never get enough of it. We can never get enough because falseness can never be verified, even if you put the full force of the universe behind it. So it's an endless cycle that can't work. It sort of seems to work because we all play the game to get along, but ultimately it cannot work. *'No reward of your Father'*, means just that: It doesn't work.

We usually can't be totally ourselves in our everyday interactions. We know full well what the results would be. Being polite and not saying what we really think or feel is so much how we live, that it is the accepted standard. The way of our world requires that you be politically correct and that you create a certain facade about yourself, which means that our artificial self-image is only necessary so that we can falsely interact with one another.

But that's what's changing in the world. So to get back to that secret weapon: Since the fatal flaw in the system is the fact that we do not acknowledge the falseness, that's all we have to do. Acknowledge. Acknowledge the falseness within ourselves and everywhere we see it, and with everyone who wants to participate in the fun. Have a big party and laugh about it all. As the grand finale of the celebration, we can thank each other for playing these parts so well that we could have this unique experience.

And the good news is that we are already doing this; the party has already started. Honesty is increasing rapidly everywhere. Of course, most people, who have trouble with conformity and see through it all, usually get themselves into trouble, but it's a start. It might not look like it on the surface, but these people are going somewhere. They become critics or comedians or just drop out of the system, but they are making a statement. Dropping out of the system doesn't help anybody and what can *I* say about being a critic? But comedy is a very good alternative. It is one of our best tricks as a means of coping with a false world. A lot of people joke about the things we do as a release, and it is often the only way to express truth and still stay out of trouble. Stand-up comedians perform a very good service because most of their material comes from everyday events and situations that we can all relate to. We laugh at ourselves in a controlled and safe environment otherwise our false world would drive us completely crazy.

But ultimately, all we have to do is remember that we don't need a self-created, self-image at all. We were born with an image that can't be improved upon. I think I mentioned in that big therefore we just covered that I have trouble with the concept of improving on perfection. We were born with a perfect image and as we stay focused on that, the way of the world loses its appeal.

Every child is born with the knowledge of having been created in God's image. It simply is not possible for a child not to know this. It comes with the territory. To become unaware of that heritage takes major work that only the influence of a world with a long history of fear could accomplish. Therefore, what we are doing here is not a process of learning about ourselves, rather, we are going through a process of undoing the falseness that we adopted as children - that falseness that we adopted for countless generations.

But all this can be easier to understand and work with when we accept the simple fact that we live in fear. I have mentioned fear before, but I am sure I didn't do it justice. What we need to realize is that we have allowed fear to become an all-pervasive force. Worse, we have allowed it to become our motivating force. We don't notice it for what it is because we are so used to it that it has developed into the accepted standard. It might not look like fear is the dominating factor in our lives because we do such a good job of hiding that basic fact. But if we were to look closely, if we were to really look at our everyday concerns with an honest and critical eye, there is only one conclusion to come to: We live in fear. And the main reason we don't see it is that we have no other model to look at.

Again, let's remember that getting into the state we are in was a very gradual thing and that in that very gradual and long process we redefined ourselves. And it's that definition that causes all the trouble. We have done a complete about-face. We have redefined ourselves and we now believe ourselves to be less than perfect. As if our very nature was flawed or even evil. Now we've gone too far! Enough already! How could the universe function or how could anything work or how could God get anything done if evil was a component of creation? Yes, we have created evil by our mistaken concepts, but evil does not and cannot exist as a basic part of reality. That concept is ridiculous. Everything would collapse. Let's give our collective heads a shake. That's absurd. The only reason such an outrageous concept can survive is because we never look at it. We perpetuate these absurd notions on the subconscious level because we are too busy coping with the situations we have created by these absurd notions. So let's forget fear for one moment and take that moment to look at what we really are doing:

Therefore when thou doest thine alms,
do not sound a trumpet before thee,
as the hypocrites do in the synagogues and in the streets,
that they may have glory of men.
Verily I say onto you,

They have their reward.

When we start to see what we are doing from a higher perspective, we will see the absurdities that have resulted in our redefined/self-defined sense of self. The above example is obvious. It is laughable now to imagine anybody announcing his intention to show what a good person he is by actually blowing a trumpet to first get everybody's attention before he does a good deed. But we can laugh at that all we want. Guess what? We still do these things. The things we do now are much more subtle than sounding a trumpet, but that only means that we have gotten a lot better at managing our false selves. It does not mean that we have actually seen through ourselves. It does not mean that we have understood why we have this need to be noticed.

But it does mean that it is time to wake up to the simple fact that expressing that need doesn't actually accomplish anything. *'They have their reward'* means that nothing else can be expected. And it means that the only reward is being noticed, which of course only perpetuates the fiction we are trying to get beyond. Giving for the sake of nurturing or otherwise attending to that false sense of self only enhances that false sense of self.

But when thou doest alms,
let not thy left hand know what thy right hand doeth:
That thine alms may be in secret:
and thy Father which seeth in secret himself
shall reward thee openly.

There is much, much more to giving than meets the eye. For sure there is a lot more to giving than making a display of it. Actually, when it comes right down to it, making a display of giving is just the opposite of giving. It's taking. Any attempt at supporting a self-image is an attempt at attracting something to oneself. And yes, we are fully capable of allowing ourselves to believe this opposite in the state we live in. The only thing that giving for the purpose of being noticed shows is that at least the concept of giving has not been completely forgotten. Even in the condition we are in, seemingly separated from our source, a part of our real nature comes through. Granted it's very distorted, but it does represent the truth trying to get through.

Having our attention on the outer world is very understandable given the state we are in, but it gets us nowhere. And it gets us nowhere because the outer world is the effect, not the cause. There cannot possibly be any real power there. Cause comes from our inner world. To activate cause, to get what we want, we must get in touch with cause.

So this is the first of those barriers that are in the way of the expression of our perfection. We quite naturally forgot the real definition of giving during our state of separation because, and also quite naturally, we are too needy. How could we not be needy in this state we are in, this state of separation from our source? Giving is one of the great laws of the universe. Real giving starts after we have released all that is between us and the source of all giving. When we get to know our real selves, giving goes without saying.

And that's why we had to do some preliminary work just to get on topic. And that's why we had a lead-up about giving and Love before that big conclusion about our perfection. And of course, giving was covered in the Beatitudes. The attitudes for being are all about developing an attitude towards giving. We just got more specific in these more recent chapters. Giving is what we are all about. So we covered it in the beginning and it keeps coming up in everything we are doing here. Giving is fundamental to our nature. Giving is how creation comes about.

But we can't possibly understand the full meaning of giving in our present state. As long as we are separated from Source and do not have our own needs met, how can we understand giving? How can we give what we do not have?

Yet our real ability to give is unlimited. As I pointed out just back a bit, infinity doesn't have a supply problem. And since we are the thinking part of infinity, we are quite naturally the dispensers of infinite supply, which is giving. Therefore, giving defines us. Making a display of giving actually points out an inability to give.

Giving has to do with co-creating with God. That's how and why giving is synonymous with our real nature. And that's why we dealt with the tough parts like going with him twain and loving your enemy, first. That was just so we could get the concept of how things work. Giving involves Love. And it involves Love with no conditions. The nature of Love is to give. Giving has nothing to do with making ourselves look good. And that's why I've been going on and on about how this self-image thing is such a stopper. Until we get back to our true image, we can't really understand enough about ourselves to see that giving is built into our very nature.

All possible needs are a given. Once we get to know ourselves again and become aware that all needs are being met and always readily forthcoming, there will be nothing to do but give. Giving is a key component of our job description. God couldn't handle giving everything infinity has to offer and that's why He created us. So that we could at least make infinity look worthwhile. A few billion people giving all they can think of should help a little towards getting infinity on the road.

I like to stop once in a while and remember what we are trying to do here. We need this detail but we don't want to get bogged down in it. We are trying to get reconnected. Giving is a part of that great road back, but it has to be real. Giving cannot be understood, let alone put into practice, when our own needs are not being met. Most of what has been covered in this chapter has been about releasing that image of ourselves that doesn't work and does not fulfill our needs. And the simple truth is that when that which has been blocking truth is removed, everything automatically flows again. When we get that, the rest falls into place. When we get reconnected to reality again and find all our needs met with ease, giving will be as natural as breathing or obeying the law of gravity.

Giving is what we are all about. There is no hardship involved. Giving is the fun part. But all this will become clearer as we go along. For now, be it known that understanding the real nature of giving is one more key to understanding ourselves.

Chapter Nine

TO BE OR NOT TO BE

*And when thou prayest,
thou shalt not be as the hypocrites are:
for they love to pray standing in the synagogues
and in the corners of the streets,
that they may be seen of men.
Verily I say unto you,
They have their reward.
But thou, when thou prayest,
enter in to thy closet,
and when thou has shut thy door,
pray to thy Father which is in secret;
and thy Father which seeth in secret
shall reward thee openly.
But when ye pray, use not vain repetitions, as the heathen do:
for they think that they shall be heard for their much speaking.
Be not ye therefore like unto them:
for your Father knoweth what things ye have need of,
before ye ask him.
After this manner therefore pray ye:*

*Our Father
which art in heaven,
Hallowed be thy name.
Thy kingdom come.
Thy will be done on earth, as it is in heaven.
Give us this day our daily bread.
And forgive us our debts, as we forgive our debtors.*

And lead us not into temptation, but deliver us from evil;
For thine is the kingdom, and the power, and the glory,
forever.
Amen.

For if you forgive men their trespasses,
your heavenly Father will forgive you:
But if you forgive not men their trespasses,
neither will your Father forgive your trespasses.

    I drove a dump truck for a bit. It had a trailer but it was not referred to as a semi-trailer. We have all kinds of exotic names for the many types of trailers and all their combinations. This dump truck trailer is referred to as a pony, meaning among other things, that it is a separate unit. That's not at all important except that to get at the point of this story I need to explain a part of the necessary mechanisms of a dump truck.

    An important feature of a dump truck is the device that opens the tailgate for unloading. A hydraulic system raises the box, the tailgate opens and releases the contents. I had observed the mechanism in question on a dump truck without a trailer and was aware that it consisted of a simple piece of equipment controlled by air pressure. The truck has air for the brakes anyway, so it is easy to install an airline to a cylinder and have it controlled from the cab.

    So I was curious how this was accomplished for the pony. Of course, I realized that an airline could be installed to the back of the pony but that seemed like a lot of additional expense and inconvenience. There are already two airlines, an electrical line, a hydraulic line, a safety cable, and a reach with a hitch, connecting the trailer to the truck. And given that all these things have to be disconnected each time the trailer is required to be separate from the truck, it would be nice to be able to avoid an additional airline for the tailgate. And that's exactly what had been accomplished and I was suitably impressed.

There was an air cylinder to open the tailgate of the pony all right, but it did not necessitate an additional airline from the truck. The trailer already has an air reservoir tank for the brakes and there is already an electric cord for the lights. The air was tapped and connected to a cylinder and the electric cord was utilized to send an impulse to the air cylinder. The electric impulse activated the air cylinder, but it was the cylinder that accomplished the actual opening of the tailgate. The entire mechanism was called, quite appropriately, 'electric over air'. Efficient, easy, and handy.

Why would I tell you this? Well, it's not because I want to bore you with the many details of a particular occupation. I made this story as concise as I could. If I thought anyone reading this would put it to practical use, I would have had to use considerably more detail. No, I tell this long story because I want to make a point. It's not easy to understand the workings of spirit because we don't have the concrete evidence before our eyes. We are by definition dealing with something abstract. Therefore, I will create a metaphor with whatever I can find.

I was intrigued by this 'electric over air' device because it reminded me of how spirit works. I can actually see an air cylinder function. I can observe the movement and be aware of exactly what it does; I can observe that the air cylinder is attached to a hook, that when moved, renders the tailgate no longer securely attached to the box which allows the tailgate to open. And more, I can understand how air is compressed and contained and used as a force to activate anything it is attached to. And this is not bad for someone who was voted the least mechanically inclined of all known truck drivers.

But even by stretching my abilities to comprehend this procedure, and by accepting the fact that there are many people for whom this little trick is quite elementary, that still leaves me with something that is not concrete and that I have to trust: Electricity. But I know that it works because I see the results. I can't see air either but I am more familiar with it and I trust it completely. The wind reminds me of it; breathing reminds me of it. I appreciate air. Also, I have been on the receiving end of electricity in an unpleasant way which put it into sharp focus for me. I take air for granted and electricity is very real to me. But even though I can't see either one, they are close enough to be concrete for me. I accept them as part of my physical world.

So how big of a leap from this is it to accept spirit and the workings thereof in my life? Results. That's all I have. Does it work? I am asked to believe that by changing the contents of my mind, I activate a mechanism that affects changes in my physical world. The only thing I have is results. I 'watched' electricity activate an air cylinder. Can I 'watch' spirit activate the events of my life? With a little practice and observation, yes, I can. The connection can be made with simple observation and from an understanding of cause and effect. A very practical thing, spirit. I don't know how we can get along without it.

But I want to get back to that concept of 'electric over air' for a moment. The feature that got my attention from the start is that the tiny amount of power emitted by the electric current activated the much larger power represented by the air pressure. I was intrigued that small power had command over bigger power. Such a simple mechanism really - certainly couldn't be called high tech, but it employed a very interesting principle. This kind of thing is extremely commonplace and has much more sophisticated applications than the activating of a tailgate on a dump truck. At the time of this writing, signals are being sent to Mars to activate vehicles that have been made to successfully land there. You can probably see where I am going with this. Maybe we're on to something here. Maybe we're getting closer to understanding something very basic in terms of how everything works.

Could it be that that's the way the whole universe functions? How big a step in understanding is it to go from an electrical current to a radio signal and then on to the electric impulse contained in a thought? It's no big mystery that our thoughts contain electricity. Science has known that for quite a while. So it would seem that the tiny power of our thoughts has command of a much, much bigger power - the very power of the universe. Maybe it would be a good idea to learn how to use that power.

So let's go back to my tailgate mechanism one more time. A few days after starting my dump truck career, I came to a hill and reached toward the dashboard to activate the engine brake. You guessed it. I accidentally hit the tailgate switch instead. That switch did not consider my mistake for a moment. The tailgate was immediately opened and the result was gravel all over the highway. I never made that mistake again, because I instantly connected cause and effect in my mind. It had a rather dramatic impact on my memory. And in case I needed additional reminders, my co-workers were kind enough to keep this topic alive for some time with a long series of jokes about my incompetence.

We are at the controls at all times whether we know what we are doing or not. The functioning of the universe is reliable and the tiny power contained in our thoughts activates the much greater power with which to take command of our lives. That communication is called prayer. Prayer is communication with God, with cause. It is being at the controls with that minuscule amount of power emitted from our thoughts to activate the greater power.

So why don't prayers work better? Why do we often have our prayers unanswered? If it's as simple as getting connected to the ultimate power with the power of our thoughts, it doesn't seem like there should be any holdup. Well, yes it is as simple as connecting with our thoughts, but there is a bit of a problem within this fictitious state we have created for ourselves. And there will continue to be a problem with prayer until we understand the system, get tuned into, and work within the laws that govern everything.

And that's why we are redefining prayer here along with everything else. Once we understand what prayer really is and how it works, we can get back to the simplicity of connecting and being our true selves again. I can hit a switch to activate my infamous tailgate and expect it to work, and the process is indeed the very same with activating the affairs of my life. But so far, my thoughts toward the finer things to which I aspire have not worked quite as well as my tailgate. I seem to be hitting the wrong switch most of the time. It would seem that I may need a little more practice. Apparently, a connection to God requires a little more than the practice required for the normal functions of our everyday activities. There has been something hindering my connection to the power of the universe.

And that would be the solid core of the subconscious patterns I have established over a lengthy period. My present conscious desires are being delayed by what I have previously established in my subconscious. And those old patterns insist on serving me according to the instructions firmly established over a period of time. Changing the content of my mind is not quite as easy as learning which switch on the dash activates the tailgate.

We covered how our thoughts need repetition and the subsequent build-up of feeling to gain the necessary power to bring about our desires. Our every thought is effectively given clearance by the subconscious before it can connect to cause. A desire for a particular outcome is often countered by a previously installed program. The subconscious, as a clearing house, is our big safeguard as well as the big holdup. It is what prevents chaos because momentary one time thoughts simply never get cleared. If a pattern opposing a new desire/signal is found, then of course clearance is not forthcoming. It's a very simple procedure and the only possible way we could remain at least semi-functional in our present state.

Prayers sometimes do not work for the simple reason that we are sometimes sending out conflicting signals. And they do not work if we have not been able to generate the feeling required. *Only that which has been established in the subconscious and has therefore become a part of our **identity** can have the feeling and the power to connect to cause.* And too, there can be quite a discrepancy between our feelings and the feeling recognized by the universe. Namely, Love. This means there is often a question of compatibility with the cosmic computer holding things up as well. Sorry about that, but all of the above can take a bit of practice when we have been living in fiction for many millennia. Prayer is communication.

The activation of the Mars vehicle required very accurate and sophisticated communication. And we can be sure that there was no question about compatibility in all the software involved. And we can also be sure that the communication we call prayer, requires a certain quality and compatibility as well.

Most of the pitfalls involved in our communication with Source were covered thoroughly in chapter three. But there is a tricky little spot about all this that is worth repeating. Those opposing patterns in the subconscious do indeed override any and all conscious thoughts that are not consistent with, or otherwise compatible with them. But there is more than a cancellation of the conscious desire that takes place. What has been established in the subconscious is the current and prevailing power. Therefore it is that established pattern that is empowered even when a new thought is introduced. The new thought activates the old pattern because the old is standing guard ready to oppose. And in the activation of that opposition, the old is more firmly established.

And that simple fact can do more than hold us up. It is of course what keeps us going in the opposite direction to where we assume we are going. And that's how and why we often get the opposite of what we asked for. And that's why prayer and all activity involved in a change in consciousness has to be a process. The process of changing the contents of our minds invites opposition and requires an informed and determined approach.

I dumped gravel on the highway because I allowed myself to be distracted. That was the real cause of my 'accidentally' hitting the tailgate switch instead of the engine brake switch. Likewise, and on a slightly more sophisticated level, any and all opposing information in our subconscious minds are programmed distractions which limit our ability to access more favourable cause in our lives. That's the reason prayer is not always as effective as it might be and that's the reason we are redefining prayer. And more, it is the reason that prayer, by this updated definition must be in secret. There has been too much misunderstanding about prayer. This update clears all that up.

> *But thou, when thou prayest,*
> *enter in to thy closet,*
> *and when thou has shut thy door,*
> *pray to thy Father which is in secret;*
> *and thy Father which seeth in secret*
> *shall reward thee openly*

It starts and ends with secrecy because we have enough distractions from our minds without inviting distractions from the outer world. Prayer without solitude has no chance and no longer meets the definition of prayer. **'Verily I say unto you, They have their reward'**, is a repetition of what we had in the last chapter. We get the same results as was indicated with **alms**. The reward for an outward display of prayer is being noticed - nothing more.

That limited understanding of prayer can't work because no contact with cause has been made. No contact with cause has been made so we get no results.

So secrecy is required for two reasons. To start with, we need solitude for our endeavours because the very process of releasing all that is unlike our true nature is very distracting and requires concentration. These things that we are trying to release will demand attention. It's a little like cleaning out the attic. You keep running into things you forgot about but you think you might want to save. So if you have conditions from the outer world to contend with as well, what chance do you have? The outer world can only contain that which is similar to what you want to get rid of. You don't need any encouragement towards your tendency to keep what you are trying to release. The last thing you need is distraction from the outer world.

This brings out the bigger problem with public prayer. Other people don't want you to change. I don't wish to be unkind, but this is the simple truth. Other people who would engage you in such things might very well not have your best interest at heart, all unknowingly of course. No bad intent on the conscious level, but we have this unconscious thing to deal with. People unconsciously try to keep the status quo and your change can be threatening. So, they will unconsciously undermine your efforts.

There is no way out of this. Prayer is personal and private. It's as personal and private as your autonomy because that's what it represents. Each and every one of us has exclusive jurisdiction within our personal kingdoms. Privacy and solitude are imperative for such an endeavour.

Real prayer, done without distraction of any kind, inner or outer, works. Once we have freed ourselves from distractions of every kind, prayer works every time. Once our communication is clear we can't miss. When prayers are consistent with the real definition of prayer, they are totally reliable - even more so than my tailgate. A physical mechanism can fail. God cannot. Each of us is an autonomous unit, complete in every way. Whenever we do not get the results we expect, it is always because of something within ourselves, something we have command over. God / Love / cause, is the constant. The only variable to perfection is us. All prayers are answered. Our autonomy and our status as children of God guarantee that. The 'mechanism' to answer prayer is impartial because it is the absolute. It cannot counteract the orders given. When all opposing habits of thought have been released and your focus is exclusively on that which you desire without any residue of content and feeling to the contrary, all is clear for the system to bring you what you want. That understanding is the starting point and the basic requirement for success.

The 'how to' - for freeing ourselves from the restrictions we have established within - is a process and was thoroughly and conclusively covered in chapter three. ... *if thy bring thy gift to the alter...*

But there is a great shortcut to all this. The effectiveness of prayer is immediate and absolute when it is consistent with the benevolence of the universe. Once you have Love in the mix, you can't fail. Prayer is absolute when it contains the fuel of the universe. I mentioned in that chapter on Love that I had beginner's luck with my co-worker. But everything we have here clearly infers that there is no such thing as luck. What my 'beginner's luck' really meant is that I didn't know what I was doing. I was quite unaware of the great power I had invoked by the simple act of getting out of my own way. That's why 'beginner's luck' works. The absence of awareness precludes the possibility of enlisting the opposite from the subconscious. And that's also why beginner's luck usually doesn't last. It's just a matter of time before the opposite pattern will come into your awareness to do its duty. The opposite pattern is bypassed when we are unaware of it but that doesn't mean it doesn't exist. As has been made clear, established states of consciousness will faithfully insist on recognition. That's why I am adamant about using total acceptance as a bridge. Its use is imperative in the interim while we are trying to remember what Love is like.

When all that hinders has been released, it requires no effort to remember Love, to feel what Love is, and to *be* in a state of Love. The all-pervasive force of Love simply flows in as a constant stream. A clear mind 'in love' does not bring up opposition and is therefore in constant contact with cause. That's how miracles occur. When all impediments are removed, Love quite naturally moves in and heals everything in its path. That's our natural state and how we are meant to operate.

So to get back to that great shortcut: It cannot be overemphasized that Love, the great benevolence of the universe, is always capable of overcoming anything. There is no need for effort or for a long process of releasing to facilitate a reconnection. When we employ Love, there is no need to even consider all the misconceptions we have accumulated in the subconscious, let alone take on the work of releasing it all as I have advocated so many times. We can deploy Love without understanding it or feeling it. We have only to use our bridge in any and all circumstances and nothing else needs doing. This truly is the shortcut of shortcuts. With this, you hook in to God's grace, and divine harmony is forthcoming in every moment and every detail of our lives. And then, after a time of consistently deploying this great and all-conquering power, all the misconceptions we have installed within us simply atrophy from lack of use.

So why then have I been going on and on about releasing all that obscures, at least twice in every chapter? Well, that was just to get on topic and get things in perspective. We certainly do not have to acknowledge every detail of our fictitious selves, but it could be useful to get a glimpse of the enormous disparity between what we are expressing and our real selves. I wanted to demonstrate what a daunting task the clearing of the subconscious is so that we could get a true appreciation for an alternate method of healing. What does it take so that we can get some idea of the huge discrepancy between our true selves and our fictitious selves? What does it take so that we may be motivated to go beyond our normal boundaries, to be motivated to exercise this relatively tiny bit of effort? Yes, all that obscures will simply atrophy after a time of staying focused on reality, but all that obscures requires respect so that we can appreciate our shortcut as the great expressway home.

***

I did some trucking in that great country just south of us. I covered around 37 states over a period of time. I had the luxury of a cell phone. How did we ever get along without cell phones? Of course, we will ask the same question when we get reconnected to God. How did we ever get along without God? The difference is that we are never without God, even when we think we are.

My cell phone worked very well. Whenever someone from home called me, the system always found me even though the caller might not have any idea where I was. I was very impressed that this could be so. I wondered what process took place that a call could go through every state and maybe even all the provinces to find me. And then it dawned on me. That's not how it works at all. That simply could not be. No, no, what happens is that my phone sends a signal announcing our location. That little cell phone was in constant communication with the system so that when a call was placed it was almost like a local call. The connection did not require searching because our whereabouts were known at all times.

I had a small misunderstanding there until I put my brain in gear and realized that there was only one way this phone thing could work. Our modern communication works much more efficiently than my thinking first suggested and so does the universe. But there can be a similar misunderstanding about our communication with God. That misunderstanding revolves around the issue of repetition. Repetition to get God's attention is similar to my imaginings that phone signals went hunting all over the U.S. of A. and all the provinces to find me. But that's not how it works. We are in constant contact with God and God is in constant contact with us. Repetition has nothing to do with contacting God.

But when ye pray,
use not vain repetitions, as the heathen do:
for they think that they shall be heard for their much speaking.
Be not ye therefore like unto them:
for your Father knoweth what things ye have need of,
before ye ask him.

Repetition is good but it's not about getting God's attention. It's about practice. It's about practice in releasing anything unlike our true nature and it's about practice in staying focused. It does indeed take repetition to get beyond that which is in the way because of the established nature of what we are trying to release or overcome within ourselves. The misunderstanding about repetition comes with the misunderstanding of what prayer is.

The old understanding of prayer was about requesting from God in the hopes that God would bestow favour. Such a limiting view is understandable from the days of darkness from which we are emerging, but it's also understandable that it didn't work too well. Prayer redefined makes it obvious that that's not how it works. Prayers are always answered in as much as we are always in communication. We are connected by thought so we are always connected. So repeating doesn't mean that we will finally get God's attention. We have God's attention at all times. It's just that we are busy contradicting ourselves most of the time. That's what repetition is for - to release that which contradicts. We repeat because it requires a process to bring up that which we need to release. And we use repetition because it requires a process to install the truth within ourselves. The good news is that it is easy to know when you are done with the process. Your prayers will bring results.

This takes us to a therefore. And that which brought us to this therefore effectively redefined prayer. This new information informs us that, since God already knows what we needin - everything is at the ready to fulfill our needs - it is us who must work on our individual kingdoms that we may be *receptive* to what already is. This is a very important therefore: ***After this manner therefore pray ye***

There is a conclusion that we may draw from looking at what doesn't work and from an understanding of how we limit ourselves. We just had a clear view of what doesn't work. Prayer redefined has a very different approach, once we understand it completely. This means once we have it installed in our consciousness, we have redefined ourselves as well as prayer.

Our Father
which art in heaven,
Hallowed be thy name.
Thy kingdom come.
Thy will be done on earth, as it is in heaven.
Give us this day our daily bread.
And forgive us our debts, as we forgive our debtors.
And lead us not into temptation, but deliver us from evil;
For thine is the kingdom, and the power,
and the glory, forever.
Amen.

The dispatcher who facilitated my travels in the U.S. of A was and is a benevolent soul, but he insisted on knowing where I was and that I was to report in at least once a day. He had a sign in his office that read: 'If you know where you are and God knows where you are, but your dispatcher doesn't know where you are..., well, let me put it this way..., you better have a pretty good relationship with God'.

But there were times when I had my phone turned off, or I may have been busy unloading or otherwise separated from my phone. That wasn't a big deal. It only meant that I wasn't in communication with home or my dispatcher. Nor is a disconnection with God that big a deal, except that we are not in communication with home or with the necessary information to function normally.

Our autonomy allows us to shut God off. And we do that by allowing our attention to be elsewhere. God is aware of us at all times and knows where we are in all ways. That's how the system works. So if we want to get anything done, we have to make sure we have our end turned on - connected so that we can check in with home. To be conscious and present in our awareness is the on switch. That doesn't mean that you have to have faith. That comes with time. But it does mean to be present/consciously aware. This state completes the connection because God always has His end turned on.

When we refer to God, we do so for a reason. It's a reaching out - reaching for something more than what our normal terms of reference give us. We want something better to happen. It's a very natural thing to do. It comes from a subconscious knowing that there is more to us than the obvious and it comes from dissatisfaction with present circumstances. We all have some sort of belief or some kind of knowing, however vague, that there must be something better. We can never shut off the real Truth about ourselves no matter how much our busy world demands our attention, or how far away our beliefs have taken us.

The above example of prayer is a formal outline - a way to take our inner knowing to the outer and to make it real and usable and a part of our everyday lives. It's an extremely powerful tool to use. I use it all the time. It fits any problem, or situation, or occasion. It is the condensed form of everything we are covering. Also, I have found that each use brings a slightly different or deeper meaning even after years of practice.

I know that all who are reading here are familiar with this, but I would like to give you my take on it anyway.

Our Father which art in heaven,
Hallowed be thy name.

The opening refers to our source and a dimension beyond our physical awareness. It starts by pointing us in the right direction. These words acknowledge our seeming separation from God, by referring to God being where we are not. And it reminds us of the unseen dimension involved - the dimension we refer to as heaven. And it makes a huge statement about our source. The nature of God is hallowed. The strongest word we have for good. We could probably do with a stronger one, but that's the best we have in the English language and you get the idea. If we include infinite potential, infinite unconditional Love, and perfection in our definition, we're on the way to understanding.

Thy kingdom come.
Thy will be done on earth, as it is in heaven.

We have been referring to our individual kingdoms right from the start. And we have made it clear that everything in our lives comes from the constitution we have adopted within our kingdoms. And we have also made it clear that a benevolent state within our consciousness quite naturally creates benevolence in our lives. So we know that our main goal in life is to create a new and better constitution within our personalized kingdoms and that it is worth any amount of trouble to clear out the old to allow for the new. Therefore, since we know our potential, we know who we are, we know what we are, we know where we came from, we know our job description, and we know the nature of God. Then, of course, that nature is the only thing we can possibly aspire to.

And that's what those three little words are saying: *Thy kingdom come.* How are you going to shorten that up? How are you going to remind yourself of everything you aspire to or your life purpose in an easier way?

And what follows clears up any possibility of misunderstanding. The result of adopting the constitution of God's kingdom within your kingdom is joining heaven to earth, which includes the highest good along with perfection: *Thy will be done on earth, as it is in heaven.* What a beautiful little thing to carry around with you everywhere you go for use at any time. There doesn't seem to be much to say after that. Once we have God's will being done on earth as it is in heaven, what more do we want?

Understanding - that's what we want. Pure understanding makes it all real and usable and down to earth. There really is not much use doing anything unless we know and understand what we are doing. Nor would it make any sense. But I wonder if there is anything with which there has been more misunderstanding than this whole thing about Thy Will and my will. The big concern is the seeming contradiction between having free will and doing God's will.

But a contradiction is not a stopping place. It's a challenge. Contradictions challenge us to increase our understanding to the point where there are no contradictions. Or just live with something that doesn't make sense. Or give it up and walk away. But what does that do to your sanity? So let's get this Thy Will and my will straight once and for all, or we will stay stuck forever.

For starters, let's imagine a scenario where someone doesn't know what to do to solve a problem and does a little research to gain information. With that information, he knows what to do and goes ahead with the project. Now, how about that new knowing that he gained? Is it the new information that dictated his action or was his action dictated by free will? That's the whole point between God's will and your will. We have free will. But where does the information and all the resources we use with which to exercise our free will, come from?

We have the Divine privilege of allowing new ideas to come into our minds. When we need to, we can look within ourselves and find new possibilities. And from these possibilities, we may choose and decide what to do or believe. That's free will. So whose will is being done in that little endeavour? We tap into the source of our being to exercise free will. God wills that we have everything we need with which to make optimum choices. We have only to be tuned in, to exercise free will.

Getting tuned in again is what this whole thing is all about. Thy will or my will is not the problem. Are we choosing from that which is given us, or are we not? – that is the question. We need to be tuned in and go from there. There is no suggestion of any kind of conflict or opposition in wills or even a hint that we have to sacrifice our will in any way. *No, what we are saying when we make use of this prayer is that we desire that God's will be done because of the **absence** thereof.* And if that's not good enough, please let me explain further:

THY WILL AND MY WILL

I like sitting in the sun. Sometimes on a sunny day, especially if we haven't had sun for a while, I sit and read outside most of the day. I have noticed that the sun appears to move across the sky during the day. That movement causes me to make moves. As the day progresses, where I was sitting earlier becomes shady. I move my chair and even change locations from the front to the back of the house so that I can stay in the sun. I do this cheerfully. I do not resent the sun's incessant movement across the sky, rather I conform to it. In other words, I am obedient to a will greater than my own, and quite happily so. I have free will. I don't have to move. I could stay in one place all day and complain about the sun's movements, but I don't. I exercise my free will to conform to the rotation of the earth on its axis because it pleases me to do so. The sun, the earth, and I get along just fine and I reap the benefits. I'm not sure if this arrangement pleases the sun but I rather think it does. So we have universal harmony happening here - so simple really.

That's an example of Thy Will and my will. Certain things are set in place so that we can function - like the law of gravity. Gravity will drop us whether we agree with it or not. And likewise, the law of Love will allow you to fall flat on your face or your head if you work without it. Yes, we have free will, but it might be a good idea to cooperate with common sense and notice how the universe functions and become aware that there are certain things already set up to make things easy and that the only way things can work is if we all pull in the same direction.

It is impossible to lose our free will. That was a gift. So when we are praying - '*Thy will be done on earth as it is heaven*'- what we are doing is working towards *restoring* our free will. We give up free-will whenever we let false and limiting beliefs control our lives. There is a fine point here that is all-important. We have so much free will that we can work outside of God's terms of reference.

But there's more:

The only reason we aspire to have God's will done is because it is not being done. We will to have God's will done on earth as it is in heaven only because of the absence thereof. But we also will to have God's will be done because there is no other will. When you have successfully adopted the constitution of God's kingdom into your own kingdom, you have effectively activated the Will of God. You have willed to have God's will be done on earth as it is in heaven. Therefore, and at that point, your will and God's will are one and the same. Do you see? Such an important point. Back up if you have to. Turn this around and play with this until it makes sense. It's worth any amount of trouble to get this.

But if we really want to get into this and take up the challenge head-on, we can take this a little further and look at the concept of obedience. How can we be obedient to God and still exercise free will? Isn't that the major stumbling block? Who doesn't rebel against the thought of obedience? Obedience in the everyday world can have rather negative connotations. There seems to be endless things to which we are compelled to conform, or that we must obey. As children, we had to obey our parents and as adults, we still have to obey endless rules at work or with traffic laws - not to mention silly, absurd, and nonsensical rules. We are always being told what to do and often find ourselves obeying rules that we know can't be right. Is it any wonder we struggle with the word obedience? The final irony of it all is that we usually end up being obedient to that which is not in our best interest.

So we seek God and again there seems to be a suggestion of obedience. Where is free will? Well, what were we expecting? We are on tricky ground learning about spirit while trying to establish a new paradigm. Tricky yes, but not complicated. There is absolute simplicity in all this. The simple act of turning our attention to God is being obedient to God, just the same as my obedience to the sun as I move out of the shade. Obedience in spiritual terms is quite different than obedience in the everyday world. When we are obedient to man-made laws or rules, or just obedient to the pressure to conform, we are acquiescing to control by mass belief or to someone who has no way of knowing any more than we do, and in fact, probably knows less.

Our inner knowing is always immensely superior to anything in the outer world. There's where our problem is. We naturally take exception to that which we know deep down is wrong. We have a subconscious knowing that the ways of the world are not consistent with free will and we feel rebellious to that from within. We take that rebellion with us in seeking the Divine because we have had it up to our ears with obedience. Too bad, because obedience to Divine will is really obedience to ourselves, and it would be the one time when obedience - if you want to call it that - would be appropriate.

But the whole concept of obedience, Thy will, my will, and free will, is easier to understand when we understand our minds. We do in fact demand obedience from our minds all the time. We train our minds to do certain things at certain times or in a sequence. Through repetition, we remember to lock the door when we leave home. That's obedience. The mind is faithfully obedient to you. Therefore you are not your mind or your body for that matter. And that's where the problem is.

We are not our minds. We have our minds serve and be obedient to us. There are endless ways that our minds serve us in the most sophisticated of ways. A skilled speaker, an artist playing a musical instrument, or someone operating a machine are all examples of our minds being obedient in very practical ways because the mind has been trained to be obedient. The mind obeys these directions. The mind faithfully serves you. But it is not who or what you are. We only get into trouble and misunderstand the concept of obedience when we *identify* with our minds. You are a Divine child capable of all things, complete with a very sophisticated mechanism/manager to oversee all things - the mind that must receive direction from you to function properly.

Therefore, the trick is to identify with that part of you that directs your mind and to appreciate all those fine details your mind attends to so well. Your mind does a superb job, but as wonderful as it is, it's nothing compared to your real self to which your mind is obedient. Your mind is only your resident manager.

This takes us back to that fiction again: Your mind tries to manage your life within the terms of the fiction it was forced to adopt. That can't work. The mind is indeed obedient, but it has received false information and it can only be obedient to the information and direction it has received.

So I hope that settles the problem of obedience once and for all. You are only obedient to yourself. Take a look at a bad habit if you don't believe me. A bad habit is only something you have directed your mind to obey and keep repeating in perpetuity or until you counteract the order. The only reason we get into trouble is that we have obedience backwards. Old erroneous programs and false beliefs demand our obedience and we acquiesce because we don't take it to the conscious level where we can do something about it. Or we just plain can't be bothered to change. And after some time, we identify ourselves with our erroneous ways.

We have then become obedient to our minds instead of ourselves - the self who directs the mind. This means that a long-entrenched habit will have emotional attachment, making change a real problem. That kind of obedience makes us susceptible to the things of this world, the very things we are trying to get beyond. Granted it may take a bit of work to reclaim your command, but who cares? There is nothing else worth doing.

So free will and autonomy are alive and well. What a relief to know that we can include God in our lives and still keep our free will intact. Mind you, one wonders what could be wrong with God's will that could make us afraid of, or otherwise unwilling to deploy it, especially when you compare it to obedience to the limited ways of the world.

All we have to do to be truly comfortable with all this is to accept the real truth about ourselves - the simple truth that we are one with God. We are that part of God freely exercising Divine will to do what we choose in this physical realm. That's the part about ourselves that we have forgotten and is what gives us all the trouble. We are One. We came here to activate divine will that Thy will be done on earth as it is in heaven. Everything already is. That's what *'as it is in heaven'* means. What we are trying to do is bring into physicality that which already exists in spirit. And we do this so that we can see and work with what is, in a tangible way. We do all this so that that which exists in spirit can be seen and understood. So that we can see what we are creating and then work from there and grow and make changes if we want to. What we are really doing is living in this powerful physical realm so that everything and anything we wish to learn or work can be easily understood - so that we can see and feel the results of what we do. That's the whole idea of the physical universe and why it has been created. It was all put in place for us so we can learn to express our Divinity - like playdough we give to children so that they can mold the things they imagine in their minds into something they can see. It's called creativity and it's what we are all about.

So maybe we can find our real purpose while we are at it. We don't have to worry about will anymore. We've covered that and we've covered obedience. And above all, we know that our autonomy is absolute. It is our supreme feature. And it's also clear that we are here to act out in the physical from the potential that exists in spirit. Spirit is and has everything we need and from which we may choose with infinite variations and possibilities - chose to activate in our playground in this physical realm for our enjoyment and learning.

Well then, since everything is already provided and we have total freedom, the only thing we could possibly be concerned about is whether or not we are in fact expressing in the physical that which we already are in spirit. We are here to experience in a more dramatic way that which only physicality can bring into focus. This experience and expression is called being which is how we came to be called beings. We are called human beings because we came here to be. Our purpose is to express and to experience and to be. That's the true and ultimate meaning of 'thy will *be* done on earth as it is in heaven'.

So what is there to worry about? Nothing. Everything is provided and in place. The only thing we have to do is be. As human beings, our whole purpose on earth is to be. It is that simple. Hardship was never part of the plan. What would be the point? Why would God create hardship when He can create anything and Love is what God is? It's us who have had a big misunderstanding and missed the point of our purpose by letting our attention wander everywhere except to the source of our being. But as we get back on track by focusing on reality, everything boils down to one question. The only question we are ever really faced with is: Are we being or are we not? Or are we so busy with made-up concerns that we have forgotten to just be? Thy will or my will or obedience or may I do what I want, are not legitimate questions at all. In our state of separation, we ask the wrong question. We ask in terms of our misunderstanding. And we've had a huge misunderstanding about our purpose and what we are and with just about everything about ourselves. We came here to *be* in the physical, what we already *are* in spirit. Being is supreme in this physical world. Therefore there can only be one question for Divine beings expressing in tangible physical forms:

'TO BE OR NOT TO BE', that is the question. I didn't make that up. That's been around for a few hundred years. We are human be-ings. The only question, based on the Truth of what we are and the expression thereof, has to be centred on being. That's where Shakespeare was going when he wrote that famous line and added, 'that is the question.' That famous line got famous for a reason. Funny how certain sayings stick even when we don't know the full meaning behind them. Are we being? *Consciously* being that is. If we are not conscious of being, we are not, for all practical purposes, actually being. Above all, we are *conscious* beings. 'To Be or not to Be', is indeed the question. Yes, that is *the* question, but it is also *the* answer - the answer about our purpose. Our purpose is to be. The answer is contained in the question.

So all of a sudden everything makes sense when we ask the right question. Since being - expressing ourselves as physical beings - is our purpose, and since the self we wish to express already exists in spirit, well then, of course, everything for that purpose is provided for. **'Give us this day our daily bread'.** That's the mainstay of our existence for the purpose of expressing what we are. That covers everything. As children of God, we are given everything we can possibly need so that we may do what we will on this earth. Give us this day our daily bread is part of the logical implication contained in ***Thy will be done on earth as it is in heaven***.

Everything is provided for, that God's will may be done on earth as it is in heaven. All we have to do is remember who we are and what our purpose is. And as we redefine ourselves and gain the ability to see where this is all going, the simple fact that everything is readily forthcoming makes sense. That's what that little sentence above means. And notice it's a demand, not would you please. We demand because it's already been given and we demand because there is no other way to activate. Everything is in place. That's why it's written 'this day.' Everything is ready to go. What we need is here now because the means of creation, complete with the fuel, which is Love, is all in place. So give us this day our daily bread is easy to say and expect for anyone who understands the whole picture. It's a given.

But without this knowing and understanding, there cannot be free will. As mentioned, we have given up our free will. It is what we are getting back to. We gave up our free will by allowing ourselves to forget who and what we are. Without that knowledge, we left ourselves in a situation where our choices have been extremely limited. We took a few little detours and created a few unnecessary problems but that's where the next clause comes in:

And forgive us our debts as we forgive our debtors. A way out of our problems is provided. Forgiveness is built into the system because we are expected to make mistakes. Making mistakes is not that big of a deal. Even the most horrendous misdeeds are forgiven because they are only misunderstandings. Such things cannot and do not have a permanent effect on who and what we are.

I recently made a serious error with my computer and it seemed to have caused a problem that could not be fixed. But no, modern technology to the rescue - one more time did technology replicate spirit. With a little advice and help, I was able to 'tell' my computer to go back to a previous date – a date previous to when I had made the mistake. And behold a miracle: The mistake was erased. Such a wonder. My computer had retained a memory of a time when it was working perfectly and reverted to that program. I was 'forgiven' my mistake. Yes, it is that simple. Where do we suppose we got the idea from? If we had to keep our mistakes in perpetuity, the universe would fall apart.

But we do need to understand how the system works so that we can activate the original program of perfection. And of course, it doesn't happen by itself because we are at the controls. I'm the only one running my computer and I'm the only one in control of my life. It is I who must activate forgiveness and the method is simple. Put forgiveness into activation by forgiving. The universe is user-friendly. So much so and so simple, that we could miss it because of that ease and simplicity.

If there was only one person in the universe then of course you would only have to consider yourself. It would be kind of lonely mind you, but you would never have to worry about forgiving anyone else. But that's not the way it is. There are a whole lot of us and so we more or less have to agree on how to do things and we need to clean up as we go along; otherwise, the mess gets so high that after a while you can't move anymore. And since none of us really knows what we are doing, we are going to make mistakes. Those mistakes can hurt someone else. Too bad, we don't really mean to, but it happens because we are all in this together. Who knows what any of us will do through misunderstanding and the resulting confusion or even anger. So there needs to be forgiveness.

But forgiving and receiving forgiveness is not making a deal. It's not like if I do this for you then you will do this for me. That's not quite how it works. Nor is it like God sitting around waiting until you forgive before he decides to forgive you. Forgiveness is already in place. Just like our daily bread. But also like our daily bread, we have to demand it. It has to be activated, and we free-will beings must do the activating. That activation process moves through whoever is doing the forgiving and wipes out error on its way. It's an automatic process. And of course the bigger the issue you are forgiving, the bigger the power that flows through you with its cleansing power. In other words, the one, or ones, you find the hardest to forgive will yield the greatest benefit to you through forgiving. And you can be sure that anyone with whom you are having difficulty represents precisely what you need in that moment. That's what that part about loving your enemy was all about. There is perfect balance in the universe.

The bible I happen to have contains these words about forgiveness: *'And forgive us our debts, as we forgive our debtors'*. But my earlier memories are of reference to trespasses; *'forgive us our trespasses as we forgive them that trespass against us.'* Maybe that's clearer because we do indeed trespass on someone else's kingdom, and whatever we do doesn't have Love in the mix. Either way, Love is the only power there is, so anything that is not of Love incurs a debt because it is taking something away - it's a minus. Love is the plus - the fuel of creation. So the only way we can get rid of our minuses is by getting back to Love which is giving.

And as has already been pointed out, in our natural state giving goes without saying. Giving is what we are all about as co-creators. Creation is the process of expressing the potential of the infinite, which is giving. Creative expression brings about that which did not previously exist. Creative expression is a gift, which is Love in expression - which is what we are. So anything that we express that is not of Love is not creative and takes something away from our purpose and takes something away from our very nature.

So anything that we create that did not come from Love needs to be attended to so that we can get back to our purpose and back to what we are. And there is a provision in place for that. It is forgiveness. It is the way to get back to our nature by remembering that we are for-giving. Therefore, forgiveness is the key and the necessary activity to getting back on track. And the keyword in the process is, 'as'. Everything is in place, so 'as' we forgive, giving is restored. God's will is re-established. As we give, giving takes place. When we forgive, we indicate that we have remembered our natural state of giving. We are for-giving. We have returned to a state in which we are in agreement with how creation functions. We declare ourselves to be in favour of giving.

And lead us not into temptation, but deliver us from evil: We always have a choice in every moment. All we have to do is *think* about what we are doing in every moment. Taking our thoughts and activities to the conscious level means being present. Yes, that can take a bit of practice but living is a learn-on-the-job kind of thing. Rehearsal is always a good idea. But that's where prayer comes in, and that's why prayer requires solitude. We need practice so that we may have the presence of mind to hold to that which we aspire when we are doing the real thing - when we are out there amid the strong influence of the world. The world around us is full of temptations that would indeed 'lead us'. But this is not where we want to be led. We've been away from reality for quite some time now, so the whole world is full of misunderstanding and habits that we would be better off without.

There is a powerful pull to the mass influence around us. The strongest pressure is to go the way of that which has been established. But we have a choice. We have a choice to conform and react, or to choose truth and Love whenever we want to. The latter choice is harder of course because it's not the prevalent influence, but that's our challenge. We can stay the way we are or we can make changes and that's a moment-to-moment thing. Holding to the ideals suggested here does indeed deliver us from evil. And that's what we are implying, and that's what we are reminding ourselves of, with those few words. That short phrase is meant to remind us of where we are trying to go.

Doing things the way we always have is the easiest. It is what we normally and subconsciously accept by default. To react to everything around us is temptation. But with practice, we can make a different choice. In each and every moment we have the opportunity to release what doesn't work and remember the truth. Each remembrance and practice strengthens the new and allows the old to atrophy. It is a process, but that's the great beauty of this prayer. It only takes a moment to run it through our minds as an alternative to reacting to the normal difficulties of life. We are at the controls. We may take command of our lives anytime we want to. With practice, we can get it right every time. That's what is meant by 'watch and pray'. It means to be alert enough to take that split second to direct our attention to real cause - Love - rather than react.

So there it is: Our daily bread, forgiveness, and the challenge of the influence of the world. Three simple and extremely concise clauses that together imply the even more concise: *'Thy kingdom come, thy will be done on earth as it is in heaven.'*

This takes us full circle: *For thine is the kingdom, and the power and the glory*: The all-pervasive benevolent force that attends to every detail at all times. We must communicate with it and summon that force to bring about heaven on earth.

Forever.

The constant, unchangeable, and eternal perfection to which we aspire.

amen

An understanding of Thy will, my will, obedience, and free will, suggests the wisdom of agreement. When we understand, we quite naturally agree/amen.

So this prayer is much more than just a prayer. It is a prototype and also an abbreviation of all we are covering. The great beauty of it is, that once we are familiar with and understand the larger explanation, we can use this prayer as a reminder - a quick little snapper to take us back to reality. Because of its concise nature, the use of the Lord's Prayer causes other parts of this sermon to flash up into consciousness. Once we have the understanding of the larger version of these teachings, this little reminder activates that larger understanding. Often one phrase, or the opening, or the conclusion will fit the moment exactly to gain a higher perspective for the situation at hand. Whatever fits the occasion best, will automatically flash up. That's the magic of this great prayer. It will bring up and remind us and therefore help us to solidify the more detailed information to which we have exposed ourselves. The Lord's Prayer is truly a priceless gift and it comes complete with the magic with which it was conceived and birthed into this world.

And here's the clincher for any leftover concerns we might have around this whole business of Thy will, my will, obedience, and free will:

For if you forgive men their trespasses,
your heavenly Father will forgive you:
But if you forgive not men their trespasses,
neither will your Father forgive your trespasses.

Forgiveness is law - the concluding definition of prayer. Our autonomy allows us the freedom to activate forgiveness and thereby free ourselves. Forgiveness is a law of the universe just like our daily bread, and or, all the other laws we have covered and will cover. It's how things work. It is how the universe is set up to function in harmony. Forgiveness had to be built into the system so that anything disharmonious could be healed. The transformation of all disharmonies is something we have jurisdiction over like everything else. We have the power to free ourselves from the limitations we have imposed upon ourselves through the releasing of it, by forgiveness. It can't be done for us. This is where individual will and Thy will and obedience are very clear. We have the freedom to activate it, or not - as we will. We are free to obey the laws of spirit or not. That's the freedom we have and our ticket to freedom. *'neither will your Father forgive your trespasses'*, means just that. It can't be done; it can't be done for us because of our free will.

Chapter Ten

TO BE OR NOT TO BE NOTICED

*Moreover when ye fast,
be not, as the hypocrites,
of a sad countenance:
for they disfigure their faces,
that they may appear unto men to fast.
Verily I say unto you,
they have their reward*

I did a bit of skiing as a child. That was a lifetime ago when we lived in the northern part of the province. Everything was very different and life was rather primitive if you compare it to how we live now. We had almost no contact with the outside world. No radio, no phone, no television - TV would have been science fiction if we had science fiction.

Skiing meant walking up hills for the pleasure of skiing down. Our skiing was mostly walking. The ratio of time spent walking to skiing was probably about 10 to 1. If someone had told me that one day I would be carried up the hill and the only effort would be the skiing, I would not have believed it. I had never heard of such a thing at the time. The thought that it could be all fun and without effort getting up the hill was a concept beyond my wildest dreams. If I could have entertained the notion, I probably would have considered it to be cheating or somehow not quite right. Earning your pleasure was old-school thinking. That old concept of not deserving lingers for a lot of us, even now. But I think we've had enough of the hardships of the past. Where did we get the idea that we have to earn anything?

It's time to update that old-school thinking. It's obvious that there is always a better way of doing things and that our modern conveniences are forever making everything easier for us. We're onto something with modern conveniences. So why not take this modern way into the process at hand. Life is a given, complete with everything with which to function. Life is supposed to be all fun. Skiing down the hill and then relaxing on a chair lift to get back up the hill, is a good example of that.

The old thinking would have us beat ourselves up with things like fasting. And that may or may not be a good idea. I wonder. But I'm sure we can take a softer approach with just a little bit of Love for ourselves. There has to be a better way that would suit our enlightened and benevolent era. I have trouble with this concept of giving things up. I have done it, but it's tricky ground. I would give up one bad habit only to adopt another that was just as bad or worse. That didn't work, so finally I decided to do it differently. I gave up a bad habit through kindness.

I decided to give up smoking. I had tripped over this quitting thing before, so I made elaborate plans to support myself in my resolve this time. I decided to replace smoking with skiing. Skiing was my reward for my efforts of giving up a bad habit.

Of course, I had skied before but that wasn't much more than standing on two slats. I knew that modern skiing was much more sophisticated and would entail lessons and cost. But my new approach immediately got me into a win-win situation. Some of the cost of skiing was off because I didn't have to fund my smoking habit anymore. And the fresh winter air helped me to appreciate breathing. So altogether it was more of a happy experience and therefore much more doable.

But replacing smoking with skiing had an even greater benefit. It appeased my subconscious mind, which is always the real problem. My subconscious was programmed to somehow not only accept smoking as a good thing but a necessary thing - shows how the subconscious mind will accept anything. It has no way of discriminating. It is a loyal servant and takes orders without question. It's not able to question - that's our job on the conscious level. So I gave my subconscious something to do. I kept it busy adopting the program of skiing and adjusting to much larger amounts of oxygen. Replacing a bad habit with a good one works.

Actually there was quite a bit more involved when I gave up smoking. I also led up to it very gradually which is something that I strongly recommend. Cutting down over a long period of time is the only way to go with anything you want to give up. Again it appeases the subconscious by giving it time to adjust. But skiing for me was a key factor and most helpful. I probably wouldn't have made it without that support I gave myself.

So let's use smoking as an example of the difficulties in giving anything up. Probably not much use to anyone who has never smoked, but you might have wondered why some people struggle and even lose the battle at times. The reason giving something up can be so difficult is that we enlist the wrath of a great tyrant in the process - a powerful opponent worthy of great respect. The mighty subconscious mind takes orders and is capable of absolutely anything once it's programmed. But that same great power is a double-edged sword. We can't have it both ways. This is part of our greatness and our power.

We put most things on automatic so that we can function. But if you tell your subconscious mind something like, 'smoke is better for me than oxygen,' which is the only way the subconscious can interpret this activity, since you are associating it with something good because it is desirable, your subconscious has no way of contradicting you. Your power on the conscious level is supreme. How else could it be? We have autonomy. Your subconscious must accept what you say no matter what. And here's where it gets tricky and this whole great power thing can backfire on you. Once your subconscious has established the 'fact' that smoke is good and life-enhancing, it will fiercely protect that program as if it was protecting your life. And you experience that as a strong desire to keep the old habit. Your subconscious mind is your loving servant, devoted to accomplishing whatever you command (and yes I know a physical dependency is developed as well and even though that is strong, it is secondary to what we are dealing with here). As I have said before, your subconscious is like a computer except that it is much, much more sophisticated and it comes complete with Love and devotion. And that Love and devotion can be used against you if you set it up that way.

Your subconscious has all that great ability, but it cannot think. That prerogative is retained exclusively for the conscious mind - our power centre. So when I had programmed this smoking thing in, which was really not in my own best interest, what I did was effectively turn my great power against myself. I had caused my greatest ally to become my worst enemy. I had caused my subconscious mind to become my malevolent tyrant rather than the benevolent benefactor it is meant to be. But by a loving approach, I was able to reverse an old program for a much more favourable result. This is a success story and typical of a modern approach that we see everywhere around us in this more enlightened time.

So while we are looking at easier ways of doing things, I want to flashback to a previous episode where I had even greater success. There is a bit of a footnote to the episode of my spectacular success with my co-worker. Let's go back to that situation where total acceptance transformed my world, where my co-worker miraculously changed into a personification of cooperation. Love had been able to do its work and affect a change only after I had released all the animosity that I had been harbouring in my mind. True, I didn't know what I was doing way back then when I had my 'beginner's luck', but I did know enough to shut up about it.

It was imperative that I remain silent about the activities, or the absence thereof, in my mind. To draw attention to what was going on with me, or to in any way indicate that I was attempting to effect a change, would have undone my good work. So of course I couldn't even consider telling my dear co-worker what had actually happened or what I had done. I could not possibly share what had gone on behind the scenes - my change in heart that had so changed the dynamics between us. Nor did he ever acknowledge the change in any way. I'm not sure if he was consciously aware of it. I rather think not. But that's not important. The point for me was that something happened that changed my world dramatically. I had a huge success by doing nothing; unless of course, you count the ability to get out of my own way as doing something. I do not know what, if any, long-range effects my change had on my new found friend, but I know that he was very different with me, and I know that my work situation improved beyond anything I had imagined possible.

We cannot change anyone else. I don't think much changed for my co-worker. As far as I could see, no other part of his world changed. He seemed to take on this personality change only with me. So what counts for each of us is what each of us does for ourselves and how it changes the immediate world around us. To have expectations that someone else will change is not part of Love. We cannot change anyone else. Yet by the use of Love, which has no expectations, people around us do change. And they do so for the very reason that their free will is never infringed upon. Our great power is that we can change ourselves and that change affects others. We cannot change anyone else, but we can change ourselves and that change magically changes everything around us.

So if it's that easy to get hooked into reality and make these kinds of spectacular gains, why don't we all do this kind of thing all the time? Or a better question would be: How did we ever get into these situations where we have all this conflict when a peaceful and productive existence is so easy? What's gotten into us that we have forgotten the simplicity of allowing natural harmony to flow through so that we may be the beneficiaries thereof? What's behind this kind of negative activity? What causes us to perpetuate situations that are clearly not in our best interest? My work experience previous to my breakthrough was nothing but torment compared to the change that took place. So, it's obvious that it would have been worth any amount of trouble to use this strategy in every part of my life forever after. Who can argue with that? Of course, we all want our lives to be better and to be without conflict or hardship.

A loving approach with myself worked with the smoking thing. And I had a lot of fun skiing. And the benefit I received with a loving approach with my co-worker was many times greater than the benefits of giving up smoking. But both stories have a little more to them. Initial success requires a little understanding to become a permanent thing:

After a few skiing lessons, I couldn't wait to tell everybody that I had taken up skiing. Other people I knew, who had been skiing for some time, invited me to go with them. They were much more advanced and I quickly found myself on hills way beyond my ability. The problem with that was that I became fearful and leaned back which is exactly opposite to what you must do. The steeper the slope the more essential it is to keep your weight forward. So I spent the rest of the winter struggling and doing all the wrong things and I stopped my progress dead in its tracks. Finally, the next winter, when another friend suggested that he and I go back to an easier place and just have fun, I agreed. We quickly learned to ski. Then it wasn't long before we took on greater challenges.

So it's not quite as easy as it would seem to affect a permanent change because of this silly business of needing attention. 'Hey look at me', cost me a season of skiing. And that same need for attention cost me a lot more than that after my initial success with my co-worker. I was not able to keep my life free of conflict or hardship even after that huge success. The big holdup was habit and the emotional attachment to the identity I had established with these habits. The biggest habit that stopped that initial success from becoming a permanent thing was the habit of keeping my attention focused elsewhere from that which would allow harmony to flow. I did not know what I was doing way back then. Skiing was very useful and I did learn a lot from it and it all ended up fine. But my greater success with my co-worker was a different thing. That success challenged my old ways of thinking and my old ways of thinking challenged my success - big time. That was on a different scale.

I had employed the limitless power of Love and didn't know it. My old habits were threatened and came back stronger than ever. I fell back into my old ways and hardly noticed it. I wasn't ready for the fundamental change involved with Love - that change in identity which is the change back to our real selves where Love would like to take us. My new sense of self allowed my somewhat hidden need for attention to come to the fore. And that need slowed my progress down to a crawl and then actually had a reverse effect. It has taken me a few decades and quite a few more mishaps to get this concept to start sinking in. I happen to know that the pitfall we are working on here requires dedicated attention. Our old ways and the ways of the world become strongly highlighted and will insist on being included when we try to make that switch back to our real identity.

But this is a happy story. A little more diligence, a little more focus, a little more sanity, and quite a bit more dedication would have served me better, but my misunderstanding, misdeeds, and mistakes would have been cheap at twice the price. Yes, I had a merry ride ahead of me that I couldn't have imagined, but even with just a glimpse of the real thing, you can never really go back.

The old pulls us back. It has to. We set it in motion to work in perpetuity. If it didn't pull us back, it wouldn't be doing its job. More, if we didn't have a mechanism within us that held strong, we would have no stability in our endeavours. We could never rely on anything or have any continuity. Life would be chaos. What we have established tends to stay established for the very reason that we may have order in our lives. That which we set in motion and maintain subconsciously is what keeps us functional. That which we have set in motion to serve us continues to serve us. It is truly a wondrous thing how the great power of our subconscious will serve us in any way directed.

As mentioned, changing how we function can be a major overhaul involving a process of acknowledging, releasing, and redoing. We surely cannot force ourselves to change. But we can change without force, which means employing Love. Everything about us and everything around us magically changes when we allow Love to flow through. Our subconscious minds will take any kind of direction, but Love is capable of overriding anything and everything.

So now that we have redefined prayer and especially on the need to do our private work privately, we need a little more emphasis because of the trap built into all this. The essential part of prayer means withdrawal from the world of everyday affairs. And that withdrawal means depriving ourselves of the 'benefits' of everyday interactions. We refer to that withdrawal or deprivation as fasting. And that kind of activity or non-activity brings out the need to be noticed even stronger, much stronger. And that's the pitfall.

When we engage in activities in what may be considered personal change, we quite naturally become quite pleased with ourselves for our accomplishments - or imagined accomplishments as would be the case at the beginning of our endeavours. And so the need for recognition will become stronger than ever. There is always the need for recognition in our state of separation as we explained earlier, but now the old subconscious, erroneous patterns will become very threatened when you engage the power of truth.

So those old patterns must therefore use everything at their disposal to try and undo your work to maintain the status quo. And what better way than where we are most vulnerable - our need for recognition. So we have this extra emphasis and repetition for a reason. A real understanding of fasting is a follow-up and completes the understanding of prayer, and more.

There is a hazard here worthy of respect and caution and diligence: You know you are doing a good thing - working on your consciousness is the best possible thing you could be doing for yourself. Well then, since this is the real thing, since what you are doing is not part of the false world - it is part of getting back to truth -how could this endeavour bring anything but applause from others?

Nice try, but that would be a very erroneous conclusion. It will have the opposite effect. Others will not applaud your efforts because it points out the limitations which these others cannot afford to have brought out. The rest of us are too busy maintaining that false image that your suggestion would undo. It takes a very strong person to look at himself and you can be sure that anyone not involved in a similar endeavour will take measures to defend himself rather than look at what you are doing. So you can be sure also, that your efforts will be undermined rather than bolstered. Even someone engaged in the same pursuits as you, will not react favourably to an outside display of your efforts. It might seem like it. But you're not inside that person's head. There is an unofficial interaction just beneath the surface in our present state that we conveniently ignore, and that is not really in anyone's best interest. That support you seem to be getting probably isn't real. This whole thing is too personal. Others are too needy and insecure. Forget getting approval or accolades of any kind from the outside world. It's not going to happen. The outside world is just not geared that way. That's our problem. If the outside world was geared to favourable support of your efforts, you wouldn't need to be making those efforts. You would be surrounded by the necessary influence and no effort would be required on your part. The ways of the world and the need to be noticed is nothing but a big hook. All it can do is keep you in the ways of the world.

      This business of maintaining a self-image can be, and usually is, all-consuming. It can occupy one's attention to the point of absurdity and still not be seen for what it is. It's probably the greatest hazard on the path back to spirit. How could it not be the greatest block back to spirit, given that the attempt to move beyond it threatens how we identify ourselves? It's mentioned three separate times in three different ways: First, getting attention with the trumpet and all that silly stuff; then praying on the corners of the streets - and now we have a conclusive explanation of the entire hazard where the need to be noticed is taken to a ridiculous extreme - '*for they disfigure their faces that they may appear unto men to fast*'.

      We have covered this self-image thing right from the start so it is no longer possible to doubt that we live in fiction. And more particularly, chapter eight has a detailed explanation of the seeming need for an artificial self-image and how that can be a real stopper. Clearly, the main cause and character of our fiction is our lack of conscious connection to our source, which is why we look to each other instead of Source for validation. In other words, that fictitious self looks within the fiction to verify itself.

So, we rebel, or somehow misinterpret or otherwise ignore information that is completely contrary to the basic way we have learned to function in this world. It is entirely reasonable to expect opposition from within ourselves when someone suggests that most of what we are doing and how we spend our time will never work. You want me to give up looking for what I need in the only place I know to look?! Apparently. That could be the reason why we have been hit over the head with this issue no less than three times, complete with dramatic emphasis.

The draw and the trap around this attention thing are subtle and strong. So much so that we tend to take that subconscious need with us everywhere we go, including our spiritual pursuits. Even in this modern enlightened time, we fall prey to this. Of course, the ways we employ to get attention now are nowhere near as blatantly obvious as the examples given in these biblical quotes, but that only makes them harder to be aware of. This hazard exists and will exist as long as we are in the state we are in, as long as we keep playing this silly game of imagining we are separate from our source and each other. It comes with the condition. It's built-in and pretty well unavoidable until we do that turnaround that is implicit and explicit here.

Our problem is that we want to incorporate the changes we encounter in learning the ways of spirit into our present understanding of who we are. In other words, we would like to enhance that fictitious self that we normally identify with. And the reason we so strongly want to do that is because that fictitious self feels inadequate, which of course it is. But no amount of enhancement will do the trick. Fiction cannot be repaired, patched up, or otherwise made real. It has to be revealed and released.

Therefore our biggest challenge is to examine how we try to get attention; although it might not be quite as obvious as making a sorrowful face. And as we get wise to ourselves, we let these things go. And that releasing leaves an opening for Source to get through which allows us to see things quite differently. We get a feeling of connectedness and a sense of knowing which includes the ability to receive what we really want. That's a change in the constitution of the kingdom that allows all good things to come through and extinguishes the need for the counterfeit forms of attention we seek from the outer world. That's the change that allows the Love from source to get through.

So of course you don't tell anyone what you are doing. You just carry that around with you everywhere you go. A serious seeker does not attract attention. You never know he's around. That's fasting. It is fasting from the normal habits of mind and activity. To speak about what you are doing or to otherwise draw attention to your inner activity is a blatant contradiction in terms. To draw attention to these personal activities from the predominant and opposite consciousness from that which you are working toward doesn't make a lot of sense. It can only undo your work.

But thankfully we are now in a position of greater understanding. As I have mentioned, we are more inclined to look at ourselves these days. And better still, we are developing the ability to laugh at ourselves and our silly games. We are becoming considerably less somber as time goes by. We are seeing through it all. And the ability to laugh at ourselves is a sure sign that we are near the truth and that the truth is near us.

Spending a big part of our time and energy maintaining a fictitious self-image really is quite funny. Especially when you consider that our identity has already been established and can't be improved on. All we can do is laugh at ourselves when we see what we have been doing. And as we see ourselves better and if we really want to get this transformation thing into high gear, there is a way.

Fasting definitely is that way. But it is time to update our understanding of fasting. Fasting usually refers to not eating for a given time and that's fine, but we need to expand our understanding to get the full meaning of it. I don't know much about fasting as it is defined in terms of not eating. I rather like eating so I seldom deprive myself in that respect. So I'm not going to spend too much time on this issue by its normal definition although I do believe it can have a dramatic effect.

So let's broaden our understanding of fasting. I have noticed that the word fasting contains the word fast. I wonder how that came about. Could it be that it has something to do with a fast way of doing things, as in a shortcut? I don't really know, but I am going to assume so because fasting by a broader definition is definitely the high road to spirit.

The key component in the definition of fasting is to refrain from, to effectively practice not doing something that we normally do. I'm sure there is any number of things we could practice not doing when it comes to the activities in our minds. Pick one - like deciding not to be critical of anyone for a certain period of time. That's fasting. A very good thing to do, but extremely personal. Can you imagine the result if you went around telling everybody what you were doing? It is self-defeating not to mention absurd. Those two activities cancel each other out and you get nowhere. So I think we can get past that one. Fasting is obviously very personal and cannot include anyone else, noticeable or otherwise.

Real fasting comes from a benevolent heart and is an occasion to allow Love to have its way. There are endless opportunities during a normal day to fast. Almost at every turn, we can choose to react or not. The presence of mind required not to react is fasting. And that's basically what is meant by **'lead us not into temptation, but deliver us from evil'**. Fasting is not doing the things that are dictated by the fictitious self. Therefore fasting is a formal way of working toward getting reconnected. Formal, because this activity, or rather the absence of activity, is a deliberate and structured way of traveling down this road we are all on. In modern jargon, it is what we would refer to as fast-tracking.

Of course the ultimate in fasting is what is referred to as meditation - shutting the mind off. It's called going within. It is the one sure way of receiving an influence other than that of the world. All things are indeed within. Meditation allows you to receive the benevolence of the universe directly. And repeated meditation causes you to establish that feeling and knowing permanently. That contact with your real self affects a complete change in the constitution of the kingdom.

I pointed out back somewhere that contemplation, pondering, etc., invite the participation of spirit and I have made a big thing about the paramount importance of thinking. And I certainly am not going to change my mind about that. If we do not employ our minds to question and imagine and try out any and all possibilities, we are truly wasting our lives.

But.

But now I'm saying don't think. There is a time for not thinking. Taking time to not think is even more important than thinking. Serious thinking about our lives is of the first importance but it's the not so serious thinking that causes our problems. It's our automatic thinking that we need to do something about. When I declare that thinking is of the highest importance, I am not referring to that incessant, obsessive chatter within our minds - that mind activity more commonly referred to as worry. That kind of thinking is useless - worse than useless, a lot worse. Real thinking comes from a basis of true understanding and that works best if we give our minds a break once in a while, which means tapping into that place where all knowledge comes from. We need to stop thinking once in a while so that we can allow ourselves to adopt a higher quality in our thinking.

Purposeful and deliberate attempts to reconnect and release compared to the slow process that takes place in the school of hard knocks can be a little demanding, but I'll take that over the hard knocks any day. And here's why: Any attempt at developing silence in our minds will bring out the negative from our subconscious. And when we discover things within ourselves that we don't want, we have an opportunity to let them go. I know. Who wants to look at all that garbage? But let's look at the alternative: Anything that is still a part of the constitution of the kingdom but that we want to be rid of, anything undesirable but unknown within us, causes undesirable effects in our lives. In other words, we create by default, through unawareness. That's the school of hard knocks. Much easier to practice what I will call rehearsal; much easier to take the time to release the negative privately, through silence, by going within, than have it come up so that you get it all over yourself. And who hasn't accumulated that which is less than desirable in the subconscious? The school of hard knocks is considered normal, but we could be a little easier on ourselves.

Time out.

If you think it's strange that I would make these suggestions to you, blatantly telling you how to run your life, I ask you to consider something else: Outside influence is the very cause of our having given up most of our autonomy. We are being told what to do right from birth. Please consider the subtle and subliminal and even not so subtle suggestions that you have been exposed to since the day you were born. There is a kind of inertia within the status quo that has great power and the ability to perpetuate itself. The direction we are given by the simple process of living in our cultural environment is extremely strong, be it overt or covert. At least I'm honest about it. I'm right up front about all of this. That's the beauty of reading. It leaves you in the natural state, with no breaks for commercials and with a clear and easy choice of what you will accept into your kingdom while you shut the world off.

O.K., we're back.

A good friend of mine made the classic comment about meditation when I brought the subject up. He said, "Meditation and I don't get along." No kidding. Of course. If shutting off our minds was easy we wouldn't need to do it. Most of us are so accustomed to living in our minds that when we try to shut our minds off, we seem to lose the very sense of what we are, which is precisely what we want to do. We're not losing much.

I have mentioned that thinking invites the participation of Spirit, but so does not thinking - and even more so. Not thinking does more than invite the participation of Spirit. Shutting the mind off allows Spirit direct access to you and allows you direct access to Spirit. It can take a bit of practice but it can also take us to a fundamental shift. And it doesn't have to be difficult if we first get into the mindset of what we are really trying to do. We are trying to redefine ourselves and we are not quite through yet.

But that's enough about meditation. I mentioned at the beginning of this topic that there has to be an easier way in our modern times. Any more on this and we would be getting into an austere lifestyle which is a thing of the past. There is no shortage of information easily available for anyone who wants to delve into this subject deeper.

But I will say this: We may get direct understanding of what we are by shutting the mind off. Incessant thinking is what overrides that sense. Only by not living exclusively in our minds may we get back to the simplicity of being. The feeling of being cannot and does not come from the mind. It's the other way around. A sense of being is what we start with and is simply experienced. That's the way a newborn starts - simply enjoying the wonder of being. But as I pointed out in the beginning, we forcibly take that away from children and insist that they develop a sense of self with the mind. And as I also pointed out, from there on, we have a fictitious sense of self, kept in perpetuity with the mind. We live in our minds.

Chapter Eleven
POWER

Lay not up for yourselves treasures upon earth,
Where moth and rust doth corrupt,
and where thieves break through and steal.
But lay up for yourselves treasures in heaven,
where neither moth nor rust doth corrupt,
and where thieves do not break through nor steal:
For where your treasure is,
there will your heart be also,

The light of the body is the eye:
if therefore thine eye be single,
thy whole body shall be full of light.
But if thine eye be evil,
thy whole body shall be full of darkness.
If therefore the light that is in thee be darkness
how great is that darkness!

    I once hauled the boom of a giant crane on a semi-trailer flat deck. The machine that this boom came from was much too big to move in one piece so it was disassembled and moved with several trucks. The main body of the machine was carried on a huge low bed and the various disassembled parts were moved with smaller tractor-trailer units like the one I was driving. We transported all of this way up a mountain to a mining site. We used an old logging road that I had never been on before which got steeper and steeper as we got further up the mountain. Finally, our destination was in sight with just a few hundred yards to go. But that last bit was by far the steepest. I needed to choose the right gear because I would be going too slow to have time to change gears. I had to make the right choice before starting up the hill. I took a good look at the hill, considered my load, and made my choice. I got it exactly right. I was quite proud of myself. The engine stayed at the proper RPM and was maxed out to the brim. My load was bulky but relatively light and the truck I was driving was modern. We had just moved up to greater power. This was new to me and I was quite enamoured with having access to that power.

I waited after reaching the top of the hill because the rest of the entourage was still slowly making it up. With nothing to do, I started checking out this modern truck I'd been given the chance to drive. I leisurely walked around it with a casual interest. But then something a little startling caught my attention. The fairly new tires didn't look so new anymore. Rubber chunks had been torn loose, leaving abrasion marks and some visible little holes. Perhaps others wouldn't notice, but it got my attention. The tires took a beating from the rocky road combined with my light load. I quickly realized that the tires would be destroyed if I were to do this continually and concluded that my choice of gear was incorrect. If I were to get a second chance, I'd use two gears lower and less RPM to reduce the torque to the wheels. In this particular situation, a lot more discrimination was called for. I learned a valuable lesson from this unique experience.

My action was an abuse of power. If I continued, I would quickly lose that power. My employer would not hesitate to assign me to a vehicle not capable of such abuse. I took the lesson seriously and implemented what I learned.

Tire damage was immediate evidence of the result of my incorrect use of power. But this business of using our God power is not quite as obvious. And the power I used to do a little damage to some tires is pretty small potatoes compared to the God-power at our disposal. Power itself is indifferent. It will lend itself to wherever it is directed. I was and am free to use the power at my disposal as I see fit, but there are natural consequences to the exercise of that freedom. I would have lost my powerful truck had I continued with my activities for the simple reason that what I had done wasn't in the best interest of the company I was working for. And just as I would have lost my powerful truck with continued misuse of that power, we stand to lose power if it is not used in the best interest of all. It might take a while, but sooner or later we will lose power. Cause and effect never take a day off and the universe insists on balance. That's the way it's set up. It has to be or it couldn't work. God is not like my employer who would take my truck away or fire me to protect himself and the company. No, that's not the way God does things, although you can be sure He protects the universe. Everything is set up so that Divine harmony will ultimately prevail. The cosmic computer never fails.

Whatever we experience is what we have activated. The system works, whether we are aware of it or not. My episode with the tires was minor and I got the message right away, so there was no real consequence unless you count the fact that I got a teensy bit wiser. But I haven't always learned so easily and nor have all my lessons been so obvious or dramatic. I have missed that critical feedback many times in my life; and therefore, missed the means to make life easy.

The thing I remember the most about my follies is that feedback always comes in threes – if you let it go that far. My tire episode was a time when I got it with number one. The first one is always easy - a minor detail to get your attention, an almost fond indulgence where you can see the loving hand of God at work. The second one is usually serious. It gets costly if you missed the feedback the first time. And the third one is a major disaster. You don't want to hear about those.

It can be said that we work for God; and therefore, we should work within the rules of the company. God certainly does not hand out penalties for misdeeds, assign you to a particular activity, or fire you. But He does provide for our every need and He does provide everything we need to function and learn.

Maybe we have a little misunderstanding on how God attends to all the details. The functioning of the details of the universe has been well taken care of. It has all been put on automatic. That's why we have such difficulty understanding why God would allow such horrendous things to happen. Those horrendous things come from us. It all comes from our free will. Horrible things can only come about when we don't know what we are doing. Our difficulty in understanding comes from the simple fact that we do not have all the facts. Yes, God is everywhere present and God is the constant: The unconditional all-loving, omnipresent, all-providing, all-encompassing, unchangeable presence - the presence referred to as the Holy Spirit. But *we* are the detail. It is up to us to keep our world running smoothly by correctly using the power at our disposal. We are the only variable from perfection while we are learning. A reason that variable got far from perfection is that we sort of forgot about the power at our disposal.

We live in a very benevolent universe. The game is extremely slanted towards constructive pursuits to the point that it takes continual insistence on destruction before we can accomplish it. But continual misuse of power will eventually get results. We can beat the odds and find ourselves in darkness if we persist.

There has to be a system of checks and balances for ultimate universal harmony and to make sure we get the necessary feedback while we are learning. And there is - or the universe could not function in an orderly way. Our mistakes while we are learning are only minor blips that quite naturally occur during that learning process. It's not that big of a deal. It's just that if our contributions are inharmonious, then a system is activated to counteract that to maintain universal harmony. It's not like God is deciding this. Or if we want to call that a decision, well then, that decision has been made a long time ago - when creation first started. There is no other way we can learn but to get feedback, even if it means tragic results once in a while. The system works, whether we know the truth about ourselves or not.

Being an apprentice - a child of God - entails making mistakes and getting the proper feedback to try it differently. Learning to work with God is a lot like learning to drive a truck. It isn't all that difficult. You just have to take the time to adopt a lot of habits that work and then keep adding on indefinitely.

I for one believe it's not a bad idea to spend some time finding out how things work and then spending some more time storing those treasures in the subconscious. And also to pay attention to the results as we go along. That's what this whole thing is about. Everything we have been working on from the beginning has been about what we need to know and about how things work. And the whole point of this little part we are working on here is the suggestion that we make sure we *store* these treasures. It's about spending time instilling these truths within ourselves. Incorporating what we have been exposed to into our consciousness defines our activities as spiritual aspirants. Our entire endeavour here is about storing these gems in such a way that they are a permanent part of who we are. These treasures in our consciousness have everlasting value. Once these Truths have become a permanent part of your kingdom, you can draw on that bank account forever without ever depleting the supply. And no one else can access the account. That's an accomplishment that is beyond and *includes* all tangible accomplishments of the physical world.

It was clear in at least two Beatitudes that the very fact that we are engaged in this activity - endeavouring to incorporate what we learn into our minds, our kingdoms - means our kingdoms qualify as *'the kingdom of heaven'*. Therefore, once we have fully incorporated these gems within; once these ideals are so ingrained that we habitually and automatically express them, we have *treasures in heaven*.

So what's wrong with treasures on earth? Nothing. Fill your boots. More power to you, as they say. Those things are temporary, that's all. The use of power without consideration of the source of our power is personal power. And that's very attractive but that kind of power keeps you away from your real power. Our real power is our connection with and our freedom to exercise, God power. So if we don't keep God in the mix, we are on a dead-end street. It's just a matter of time before we run out of gas if we carry on without a conscious connection. All the wonderful things we have in our everyday lives are fine but we need both and we need to get them in the right order. That's why it is suggested that we take the time to do whatever is necessary to make this sink in. I am convinced we can get a better deal if we make sure we know how things work. Treasures in heaven are the ultimate security.

So it comes down to attention and concentration - what you have your eye on. We get what we concentrate on. That great power we have at our disposal is capable of anything. So if we focus exclusively on what we have in the physical world to the point of ignoring spirit altogether, then we are in a big mess. I don't like the word evil, but it's probably not too strong a term when you consider the contrast between being connected and not. To turn our attention entirely to accumulating the things of this world is very tragic. To use our almighty power and ability to create without acknowledging the source of that power is to cut ourselves off from power. It misses the bigger picture completely. That kind of activity is so far away from the definition of a God being, so far away from our job description, and so far from our own and everybody else's best interest that it does require the strongest word we can find. So who am I to quibble over a word or to question the wisdom imparted here? O.K., evil it is.

It's one thing to be out of step with universal harmony but look at the consequences on a personal level. Spending full time on possessions leaves you with absolutely nothing because all those things are temporary. So at the end of the day when you have nothing else in the kingdom...., well, I find it hard to finish this sentence. *How great is that darkness* indeed?

But the good news is that the intensity of this physical world we live in is what makes permanent changes possible. The consequences of our choices are often so dramatic that the powerful emotional experience is what makes a permanent record on the soul. Therefore, we get to keep whatever we establish as a change in the constitution of the kingdom, forever. But the best news of all is this: It does not matter if a powerful emotional experience is good or bad, the result of that experience still gets recorded in the soul as something permanent and positive. The soul has no way of understanding bad since it lives only in eternal Love. So experience is just that, in greater terms, and experience is the only way to grow. All experience is simply taken in by the soul to be more of what it is. It is truly an astounding thing we are accomplishing with this business we call living. So in certain terms, we can't go wrong. But we might as well do it the easy way. Learn through high drama by all means, but that drama doesn't have to be painful – you don't have to get close to Aunt Ester's breath.

We have this greatness within us which is our potential. If we use that great power as we are meant to, it is capable of creating heaven on earth. But if our focus is away from our true definition, then that same great power is also capable of creating all manner of negativity. That reverse focus is fully capable of creating the worst situation imaginable.

The light of the body is the eye:
if therefore thine eye be single,
thy whole body shall be full of light.
But if thine eye be evil,
thy whole body shall be full of darkness.
If therefore the light that is in thee be darkness
how great is that darkness!

If our focus is exclusively on Truth, then that's what we are going to get in every part of our experience. But if our attention is on other things, that's what we get also. We can use that same great power of focus against ourselves. As Sons of the most high, complete with free will, we can do anything, including bringing about great darkness. And the fact that we don't know what we are doing doesn't change things. Ignorance of the law does not change the law.

It's very simple. The same almighty power that we possess which is capable of all good things is also capable of inconceivable destruction. An obvious example of great darkness is the events of September 11, 2001. History has many dark points. History in general is dark. So with all the power we have in our hands, it's critical that we become aware of it. More so now than ever. And again, as I have already pointed out, none of us are immune. We all contribute to the darkness. We all contribute to mass consciousness. Each dark thought even the nicest people entertain is not exempt. It contributes to the pool - that same pool that some people draw from to perform the darkest of deeds. So in that sense, we all contribute to these dark deeds. Sorry about that, but we are all in this together and to imagine that any one of us is somehow exempt from contributing to the events of the world is the first big mistake. Even anger and bitterness that is justifiable must have its effect. The law is not changeable. Hatred of a terrorist for example, even by someone who has lost a loved one as a result of a terrorist act, is still hatred and can only contribute to the negative pool. (But let me quickly add that I can't even imagine the anguish involved in such an experience and I do not in any way wish to belittle the horrendous suffering that some people in this world endure).

The law of cause and effect is absolute and has no way of bringing compassion and forgiveness to any situation. The activation of Love, compassion, forgiveness, and healing, belongs exclusively to conscious beings. That's us. We are representatives of God here on earth. We are beings of Love! Any thought that we entertain that is not of Love must contribute to that which is not of Love.

More specifically, here's how it works:

Think of the atmosphere in a place of business that you like - maybe your favourite restaurant. You probably go there for that atmosphere among other things. And the good atmosphere in that place is no accident. The people who run the business are of genuine good cheer and it shows. The people who patronize the place pick up on the feeling and add to it so that the good atmosphere is increased and kept in perpetuity with ease.

That same kind of thinking can apply to a small town, a big city, or even an entire country. Some have a good atmosphere and some do not. None of this happens by chance. The people in every example entertain benevolence to some degree or other. Even the world atmosphere is changeable and has changed. The atmosphere in the world is different now than 40 years ago. We can change the atmosphere in the world anytime we want to. But criticism of the world atmosphere is in itself a contribution to a less desirable atmosphere. Anyone who wants a better world cannot condemn the way the world is now without contradicting himself. Again, the law is absolute. Negative activity of any kind within our individual kingdoms must have an effect on the world no matter how much it may seem to be justifiable.

Our biggest problem has always been that we have not known enough about ourselves. We have been unaware of the power we exercise and the effect that it has. We have had a very inaccurate idea of what we really are. We have not known our greatness and that's what got us into trouble. But it's also what we are working our way out of.

The good news is that the Love we administer within the kingdom is many times more powerful than any slip into forgetfulness. As mentioned, the game is very slanted in favour of the house.

Chapter Twelve

THE KINGDOM OF GOD

*No man can serve two masters:
for either he will hate the one, and love the other;
or else he will hold to the one, and despise the other.
Ye cannot serve God and mammon.
Therefore I say unto you;
Take no thought for your life,
what ye shall eat, or what ye shall drink;
nor yet for your body, what ye shall put on.
Is not the life more than meat, and the body than raiment?
Behold the fowls of the air:
for they sow not, neither do they reap, nor gather into barns;
yet your heavenly Father feedeth them.
Are ye not much better than they?
Which of you by taking thought can add one cubit unto his stature?
And why take ye thought for raiment?
Consider the lilies of the field,
how they grow;
they toil not, neither do they spin:
And yet I say unto you,
That even Solomon in all his glory
was not arrayed like one of these.
Wherefore, if God so clothe the grass of the field,
which today is, and tomorrow is cast into the oven,
shall he not much more clothe you,
O ye of little faith?
Therefore take no thought, saying,*

What shall we eat? or What shall we drink? or , Wherewithal shall we be clothed? (For after all these things do the Gentiles seek:) for your heavenly Father knoweth that ye have need of all these things. But seek ye first the kingdom of God, and his righteousness; and all these things shall be added unto you.

On more than one occasion I have been asked if I have a computer. And when I reply in the affirmative, the questioner will go on to inform me of something I could access on the internet. The prevailing belief seems to be that having a computer is synonymous with having internet. That certainly is understandable, as most people who have computers have internet, but I do not. Even though I am quite enamored by it, it happens that I do not have internet right now because I want to keep my distractions to a minimum. But I think the internet is a most wondrous thing. What a concept. To be all connected with one another. Now we're getting somewhere.

It seems that when I am asked if I have a computer, the real information the questioner wants is if I have access to the internet. Now I don't want to get picky but I would prefer that the question be more accurate. Having a computer is essential to getting internet but a computer does not come with the internet. There is an additional step and a fee and so on before your computer will access the internet.

The inability to grasp this concept or the lack of clarity in forming the question is no big deal. That's just the way some of us think. So I don't worry about it too much. We all have our limitations. I, for example, have great difficulty with the most trivial mechanical concepts to the point where there have been times when others did not take me seriously when I asked for help.

So these kinds of things help me to realize that a lot of us have a similar problem with God. When someone asks me if I have a computer with the assumption that I have internet, I could just as easily ask if that person was hooked up to God since there is not much use in having a body unless you are hooked up to God. But I refrain from such a derogatory comment because I'm trying to cut down. But my impertinent question would be just as valid as the question about the internet.

We seem to somehow believe that all our needs will be forthcoming from God even though we haven't bothered to get consciously hooked up. And that's all fine except for one teensy little thing. That can't work. Just being vaguely aware of God or even keenly aware of the existence of God doesn't get you what you want any more than being aware of the internet without the hook-up enables you to access the net.

To function as we were meant to, we need to be all hooked together and to God. That's the only way we can get about this business of furthering creation. And having a body, like having a computer does indeed logically infer that we are hooked up to God and each other and that we can access any and all information so that we can work together and all have a common understanding with which to work in harmony. But there are some details to attend to, to make sure we are hooked up. Of course, we *are* hooked up or we would collapse instantly. But unless we are *consciously* hooked up, we are not, for all practical purposes, plugged in.

I did walk up my favourite mountain in all of the seasons: That mountain where I had that infamous encounter with a coyote one winter as I mentioned in chapter one. And on one very windy spring day, I had occasion to make an interesting observation from a vantage point on that mountain.

Many flocks of geese caught my attention. Not so much because my attention is easy to get, as for the fact that geese usually announce their presence in a very audible way and never more so than when they are migrating. I can only assume that there is a lot of communication going on and that this is probably necessary. I don't know what they were saying to one another but they sure were doing a good job of getting to where they were going. And they weren't just coasting with the wind. They were working at it just the same as any other time but probably doubling their speed with the help of the wind.

I noticed they were flying in formation. Taking advantage of that strong south wind and flying in a V. There were no less than a dozen flocks that day - that very windy day. There was something in the air that spoke of exhilaration and change. The wind and the geese and the changing of the season were all quite inspiring. Life! Exuberant life in expression, propelled by Divine harmony.

The geese get to where they are going because they cooperate. A lot of common understanding and a lot of harmony involved in that little endeavour. Not bad for creatures who can't think and don't have words – or don't have computers or compasses or maps. Not to mention the fact that we would have to do some very serious planning to get that many of us to work together on a certain day at a certain time of the year when conditions were just right.

So when I got to the top of the mountain, I watched for a time. They crossed the valley in record time and disappeared from my view over the next mountain. They sure seemed to know what they were doing - going straight north with that strong south wind. I wondered if they catch a north wind in the fall when they go back south. I'm sure they do.

And just now, I look up and I notice a bird perched on a telephone pole outside my window. I watched as it moved its head around, observing its surroundings. It occurred to me that there was a complete entity there - a unit of consciousness capable of navigating the environment and attending to its needs, experiencing life without a care in the world. I wondered what was going on in that brain. And then I realized that that bird wasn't thinking at all. All animals just know. There is no pondering. That bird was simply being. All animals have that ability ingrained. It defines their purpose. Since they don't have the ability to think, they cannot imagine anything other than the experience they are having. Very limiting of course but it does say something about the nature of physical experience. They have awareness; they are aware of being because being is their purpose. They are not capable of making any other choice. They make choices all the time but not as a result of weighing the consequence or pondering the wisdom of that choice. They choose to look for food or look for a mate if it's the season. Or sometimes they just play because that's what occurs to them in the moment. They are always spontaneous. They do things by what we call instinct.

We are so different from the animals that it's hard to compare. We can ponder and put concepts together and add to someone else's concept even from generation to generation until we exercise our creative abilities to the point that we can find a way to get to the moon. We are aware in a much more profound way. We are aware that we are aware and we know that we know. And from there, with inspiration, imagination, and the great ability to reason and ponder, we can do anything. We can consciously and deliberately make choices knowing that we are doing so - all because we have a conscious mind.

The animals do everything subconsciously because that's all they have. And we can run on automatic too. We can do everything subconsciously if we choose - that happens by itself when we don't make conscious choices. And that's O.K. for a lot of things, but you better have some pretty good programs in place. Like for driving a car for instance. If you're going to go on auto-pilot, it could be hazardous unless you have some good habits established.

Living life is another example. Life can be hazardous without good habits in place. That's what habits are for. Habits serve the same purpose for us as instinct does for animals. The big difference is that we program our habits, but the animals come with that built-in, evolved over a long time of trial and error. What didn't work usually costs a life and so that idea slowly gets deleted from the species. But we don't have to do it the slow or the hard way. We can examine what we have decided to do 'instinctively' and do something about it. Even the basic instincts that we are born with are under our command. We can look at absolutely anything we do and make adjustments. We can add, subtract, modify, delete, adjust, and or, completely revamp. And we can decide to do something other than what a lifelong habit would dictate from moment to moment. It's called freedom and we were born with it. Animals have freedom too, but our freedom is unlimited. It comes with the territory. We have the same freedom as the animals but with one big add-on. We have this most wonderful ability to think and with which to exercise our freedom in ever new and creative ways.

Everything we need is also provided, the same as it is for everything in nature. But again, with an important add-on. We come with more - a lot more. We know ourselves *as* beings, consciously. Therefore we can *be* anything we want. For us, there are no restrictions. Our predispositions are changeable on a conscious level. We have the capacity to change our minds and change complete programs within our minds. We are in charge of our evolution because of our conscious knowing.

So what is it that restricts our freedom? What did we do that caused us to be in this state where we are no longer free? And what question could be more important to ask and address?

Well actually, it's that conscious knowing that got us into trouble. The animals know what they need to know and not more and they, therefore, function very well and more or less stay out of trouble. We know what we need to know as well, but where we got sidetracked is with our additional knowing. What did us in is the simple fact that we know that we know. It was through this knowing that we know, that we could, and we did, commandeer that knowing as our own: Big error. To imagine that what we know comes from each separate unit we believe we are misses the purpose of individuality and conscious awareness. That thinking closes the door to any real new knowing. It stops the natural flow of the ever-changing moment-to-moment incoming information. When we started believing that our knowing was all our own, we effectively cut ourselves off from the actual source of all knowing. We did the one thing that animals are not capable of doing and to our great detriment. We shut ourselves off from our source. Yes, each of us is individual and each of us has complete autonomy. But that doesn't mean that we are separate.

That's how we lost our freedom. We lost our freedom because we cut ourselves off from the ever-new information required in ever-changing circumstances that could keep us free. We cut ourselves off from the very source of all information that is essential to free beings. We became closed circuits like closed-circuit TV. Closed-circuit TV works well for monitoring in a particular location for security reasons, but it's not hooked up to anything; you can't change the channels or watch anything else. A television set used for closed-circuit is extremely limited. But if you hook it up to cable or satellite, then its ability to display information increases by so much that you can't compare.

Likewise, once we acknowledge the simple fact that we can know nothing and can do nothing nor get new information with which to make changes on our own, we start the process of getting hooked up again. That simple act of acknowledging starts up the process. It is the beginning of opening the circuit. We start taking in a little more than that which we have adopted within our tight little unit. And then if we sprinkle in everything else we are learning here, it just keeps clearing the connection. As this process continues, we can access an ever-increasing amount and variety of information with which to make choices. And when that process of connecting is complete, we get back to our ability to access what is literally infinite information, in every moment. We get tuned into real knowing and we come back to our original awareness. We know exactly what to do at any given time to fulfill all our needs and desires - not to mention the fact that we experience the joy of absolute freedom.

Those flocks of geese I watched flying with the wind that invigorating spring day were working in Divine harmony. They are aware of the sacredness of being and everything they need was and is always provided. The geese know very little compared to us, but they do know that they are part of God in expression and they manifest that expression very well. They do not have the ability to be aware of God on the level that we can, but they also do not have the ability to be unaware of God. There is only God in expression and the geese are part of that and they serve their purpose by the simple act of being.

And we can do that too. We can serve Love and therefore serve our real nature and therefore serve ourselves by just being. But we cannot serve *any* purpose if we concern ourselves *exclusively* with filling our needs. As pointed out earlier, our supply is a given. We have concerned ourselves with filling our needs to the point of letting that concern become our main focus.

And did we notice that we have moved things up a notch and brought in a new phrase? For this, we had to rename the kingdom. For the first time, we have reference to the '*The kingdom of God.* Working on getting there is the **kingdom of heaven**. Arriving is the **kingdom of God**.

And learning how to get it right is a process - the end result of which is *righteousness;* right-use-ness. The right use of our God power so that we get results: *And all these things shall be added onto you.*

But we have covered righteousness before. There is a right way and a wrong way of doing all things. We are finding the right way and who would not use a better way when it is available? The kingdom of God comes with a whole new attitude and a whole new attitude invites the kingdom of God.

The geese I watched who were going about their business with such precision exemplified cooperation. We might wonder where they get all their information that they are able to get to their destination better than a guided missile. These creatures know what they are doing. They cooperate with nature and with one another and they get results. They are connected and know exactly what to do. They don't plan or ponder the likelihood of a wind change because they don't have that ability. They just know and do. All the information about weather and everything they need works in their favour and they just do the right thing without thinking. They are connected and have the information they need at all times because it is impossible for them not to. So of course all their needs are taken care of. Could we do the same? Yes, and more: A lot more. *Are ye not much better than they?*

Did I mention that the difference with us is that we have a conscious mind? We have infinitely more ability and freedom than a flock of geese because of our ability to make any number of choices. Yes, we can make mistakes as we go along, but that's nothing once we start getting tuned in. Mistakes are only minor adjustments as we learn to firm up our connection. The geese make these minor adjustments all the time. I think that's part of what all that honking and constant adjusting of the V is all about - although I suspect there is a lot more going on with their communication. The sounds they make are a necessary part of accomplishing something together that not one of them could do on its own. There is a constant and natural multiplication of energy and a pull towards harmony taking place as they fly. If they are making mistakes, the mistakes are minor and part of the force of natural order because they are tuned into the natural order. A lot of the adjustment is the simple exercise of taking turns breaking the wind. The energy they need during migration is so much more than that which is required in their normal activities that their accomplishment can only be described as one of the wonders of nature.

But to get back to us, if we want to take a cue from the geese, we could start with a lot less concern. We God beings - we, who are the *'sons of the most high'* - can do better than that, and certainly a lot better than we have been doing. We have everything the animals have *and* a conscious mind. We are capable of anything because of the power of that almighty conscious mind. *Are ye not much better than they?*, means that we are provided for just like all creatures but with one big important add-on.

What a luxury to be able to consciously decide what we want to do from a secure base of provision. To be able to ponder, imagine, plan, and therefore expect a certain outcome from a particular course of action. Now that's creative. What freedom. That's as creative as the Creator, which of course is what we are. Possession of a conscious mind defines us as creators since it gives us unlimited choice. That gives us pretty high status. Sons of the most high indeed.

We are connected to God through thought and so are the geese. Can anybody tell me how else we could be connected? What other means might we have to be in communication? If there was an easier way, I'm sure God would have thought of it. So why not take that ability and deliberately connect to God. Can we be thinking about God all the time? Of course; it is our natural way. We have the capacity to be thinking about several things at once and we do it all the time. And our natural state is to have God as the major part of our focus at all times.

We have a body for the purpose of being. Not to have to run around frantically looking after the body as if that is all there is to us. That misses the whole point of what we are about. No matter what we do or accomplish on our own, it's nothing like what already is:

Consider the lilies of the field,
how they grow;
they toil not, neither do they spin:
And yet I say unto you,
That even Solomon in all his glory
was not arrayed like one of these.
Wherefore, if God so clothe the grass of the field,
which today is, and tomorrow is cast into the oven,
shall he not much more clothe you,
O ye of little faith?

We have done such a thorough job of ignoring that which would direct us to optimal choices in each and every moment that we act as if these choices don't exist. We seem not to believe that everything we need is as readily forthcoming as it is with all of nature. And since we are all-powerful and we can believe what we want and let that become 'instinctual', we are capable of creating a situation where we have to work at getting our needs met. And we did. We no longer believe that it could be that easy - all we need provided without effort. So of course that's the way it is. We have created a self-fulfilling, self-perpetuating situation. And we've done a very good job of it. We have a lot of things in place that support the theory of scarcity and struggle. There is a huge vested interest in maintaining things as they are. Is it difficult to change? It can be if we want to make it that way. But it doesn't have to be. There is always an easy way. Again we can start by looking at nature. All of nature is lavish, abundant supply.

I've been talking about releasing what is artificial within us so that we can get back to our natural way of being and therefore our natural supply. That was the point of getting past our self-made limitations so that we could begin to see that our daily bread is a given.

But because we have drifted so far from reality, getting reconnected has to be a gradual thing. We can't just stop everything we are doing and expect all our needs to fall from the sky at this very moment. There has to be a process. For sure there had to have been a process that got us this far away. So now there has to be a process of changing our thinking just to get pointed in the right direction. Then the real process of reconnection starts. And then it's just a matter of time and the day will come when everything we are being exposed to here will make perfect sense. And then we will quickly learn how to do things the easy way - the way in which all needs are fulfilled as natural as the air we breathe.

Yes, getting hooked up again has to be a deliberate and conscious thing. But there is no hook-up fee, nor any ongoing charge. Once you are hooked up, your subscription is for eternity and there is no cost whatsoever. It comes with the territory. Being born is your eligibility. Okay, where is the switch, you ask? I'm coming to that. Aside from the fact that the switch is everything we have covered, are covering, and will cover in this whole endeavour, I can be a little more specific.

As things stand now we do have to make a bit of effort to get hooked up, or plugged in, or otherwise connected again. It might seem a little tricky at first, but only because we are out of the habit and have been focused elsewhere for such a long time. Once we have done a little work and adopted some new habits, getting connected is as natural as learning to walk. That connection takes a conscious, deliberate, ongoing effort at first, but once we have practiced for a while, something wonderful happens. Your practice has notified Spirit of your intention and Spirit takes over the process. You become aware in such a way that it becomes impossible to be unaware ever again. That's the switch. With enough tries, one day it clicks in, and nothing is ever the same again.

Being connected to God is all about what already is and about the way everything was set up to work. If we have any trouble getting back to that, it's because of this: Our unnatural state has become natural to us. So now the things we have to do to get back to our natural state, quite naturally, seem unnatural.

Once more with the geese: What they accomplish is truly amazing. They understand a little more than just communication. They understand the power of Love. That's their connection and the only connection there is. They understand that because they are not capable of misunderstanding. That is the natural state. Nature works. But just imagine what nature could do with the ability to think. That's us! We have all that ability to be tuned into Divine harmony, *and* we have the ability to think. We are the thinking part of nature.

In the meantime, if we like, we may anticipate how much better everything will be when we are aware of our oneness with spirit again. Although we will not really know what it is like until we are there. No matter what we say, no matter what words we use, and no matter in what way we can describe being connected compared to being disconnected, it still leaves us with a problem. It leaves us with a problem because it implies that you can measure how much better the connected state is than not being connected. But you cannot. There is no way you can compare. There is very little in the disconnected state that is anything like the connected state. Therefore the attempt to describe the condition we are seeking always falls short and is misleading. The reality we are seeking cannot be described in terms of the non-reality in which we live, just as light cannot be described in terms of darkness. The infinite potential of nature consciously directed goes beyond our present imagination.

But we just happen to have the software for the hook-up. Our true nature as Love is the universally compatible software for the great connection.

THEREFORE

Take therefore no thought for the morrow;
for the morrow shall take thought for the things of itself.
Sufficient unto the day is the evil thereof.

On many occasions, I have watched a flock of birds take off all at once as if they were one unit. And also on many occasions, I have observed what takes place when I am stopped at a red light. I have noticed when the light turns green, we each start moving only after the one ahead of us starts moving. The delay is not much but it's noticeable, and that slow start is very time-consuming in terms of getting the traffic flowing again. Yet we all have the same prompt in front of us that could facilitate unified action. The green light is the outer and obvious direction to which we could take our cue and with which to work in harmony. So why don't we seem able to do such a simple thing when the direction is clearly evident to our physical senses? Surely we can work in harmony as well as the birds.

Divine harmony is available at all times, and as if that wasn't good enough, we do have such things as a system of traffic lights and the likes if we insist on using our outer senses with which to operate. So what's the holdup? I don't think the birds have such glaring outer clues. Except for a sudden appearance of a predator and other outer signals, the birds seem to act from some kind of inner direction. Why can't we do the same or better?

I haven't noticed these kinds of questions on the table in most of my encounters with others. But then, I haven't noticed great numbers of people flocking toward me to hang on to my every word. But what if this was the kind of question that could help to point us in the right direction to begin to understand ourselves better?

Mind you if we wanted to start working on such things as leaving a traffic light in a more coordinated fashion, it would probably help if we didn't park so close to one another. No bird would ever park so close that it didn't leave enough room to flap its wings. I think the reason we stay so close to each other is because we have this sense of separation and that doesn't feel right, so we subconsciously try to make up for it. So if we really want to address this question of unified activity, we have to take a long hard look at this business of feeling separate from one another for starters.

Without dealing with this unity issue, the concept of leaving a stoplight all at once can only seem impossible if not ludicrous. How are you going to get everybody to concentrate their attention so keenly when we have all these concerns of everyday living demanding our attention? And who would be that trusting? Are you really going to start up immediately when the light turns green, trusting that the person ahead of you will do the same so that you don't run into him? So we're sort of stopped before we start on that little plan. If we were going to take it seriously that is. And that's fine and to be expected, but that still leaves us with the birds as superior to us. And then what do we do about that old expression, 'it's for the birds'?

And that was just the first thing we could bump into. If we had nothing else to do but ask this question, we would have to look at ourselves and how we function. And then we might ask a further question: What have we become that we need all this help with direction so that even with that help, we still literally bump into one another? It's one thing not to be able to leave a stoplight in a coordinated fashion but what about car accidents? I haven't noticed the birds having a lot of midair collisions.

Could it be a lack of attention? I think most of us would agree that lack of attention is a common factor in car accidents. God knows we have enough things demanding our attention. Attention? Is that all it is? Is it our attention that makes all the difference? Is it our attention that separates us from the wisdom of the birds and separates us from our own wisdom? Yes. Well then, if that's the case, what are the birds doing that makes them able to function with such precision that you would swear they were all one unit?

The birds function as one unit because they know themselves to be one unit. They are in constant communication with the particular stream of information that supplies that particular knowing for their particular species, for a particular location at a particular time. And they are in constant communication with each other. But more important, they are present.

These simple and inferior creatures are expressing God because they *are* an expression of God - so simple it's almost unbelievable. These beautiful creatures sure aren't wondering if they did the right thing by sitting in the sun for an extra half hour this morning or whether there will be a traffic jam that could cause them to miss an appointment. And that's what keeps them out of trouble.

The birds are one unit and so are we.

We consider these beautiful creatures, if we consider them at all, as barely worth our attention, and yet we function in absolute chaos compared to what they do. Maybe we don't address these real and pertinent questions about how we function, because we subconsciously know that it would reveal something about ourselves that we don't want to look at. Like Pandora's Box. If we started looking at these kinds of things, would everything become unraveled? Yes, it would. So who in his right mind would address these kinds of questions when we have real concerns in a real-world of cause and effect and alarm clocks to consider and the rent to pay?

The only answer that comes to my mind is that the only creatures capable of asking and addressing questions are people. Unless of course, all of us God beings who are capable of thinking and have unlimited ability to create as we wish, have somehow shut ourselves off or have established collective amnesia. Or could it be that we got a little mixed up along the way as we were playing? Could it be that we started doing things backward just for fun, and then forgot about it? And could it be that we got a little carried away with this little game of focusing our attention exclusively outward and have become so enamoured by the game that we have forgotten that our attention is a two-way street? Surely not. That would be absurd. I must be spending too much time alone.

Still, I find it hard to leave this attention thing alone. This whole concept of attention has grabbed my attention to the point of fixation. The first three chapters of this section were devoted to what happens when we look for attention from the world. And attention came into sharp focus again with the issue of what we accumulate for ourselves. And we ended with a major explanation of what happens when our attention is exclusively directed to getting our needs filled instead of directed to the source of our needs. So this whole section has been about how we go about getting what we want. And it's about how we are actually looking in the wrong direction. So maybe it's not a bad idea to focus some of our attention on attention.

It has been made very clear to us that our biggest problem is that we want to be recognized. Whether it's for how we appear, or for how successful we are, or for what good and giving people we seem to be, or even for how spiritual we appear to be, it's all about wanting to be recognized. And that's all fine, but no matter how much recognition we manage to get from others, it can never be enough. It can never be enough because the attention we really want cannot be replaced. Deep down, we know of our perfection and we want *that* to be recognized. But no amount of recognition from the outside world can replace our recognition of ourselves. Until we, ourselves, each of us, recognize ourselves as complete and perfect beings, no amount of attention or recognition or any and all the wonderful things of this world, and or, all the successes one can imagine in this world, can replace the recognition and validation of one's true self, by one's self.

Therefore, it's time to take the whole concept of therefore to a higher understanding. As mentioned, we must understand the statement followed by a therefore. When the therefore makes sense, it's a pretty good indication that we have understood the instruction or the explanation of the matter at hand. And when it doesn't make sense, well of course you just throw up your hands in despair. Or go back and try again.

But there can be more to a therefore than making sense. A therefore can lead to a misleading conclusion. We can go over all the material that leads to a therefore and have a good understanding of it, and still have a problem. Maybe even a bigger problem than we had before. Sometimes a therefore can get us into nothing but trouble.

For example with this particular therefore, it is possible, after a complete intellectual understanding of the concept, to immediately take action consistent with the conclusion. It might seem logical to leave an unfulfilling job for instance, based on the fact that there is no need to worry about tomorrow. With the knowledge that all our needs are always taken care of, this would seem to be a reasonable course of action.

But:

But that would not be wise because there is a little more than the obvious going on behind the scenes here:

As we know so well now, our subconscious minds insist on maintaining the status quo. And we know that the subconscious will do whatever is necessary in its dedication to you in terms of obeying your commands. It matters not what the commands are, your subconscious blindly obeys and is fiercely loyal. And most of us have a strong program of concern about our needs being met, whether we know it or not. And more, that program will not be deleted by the simple act of reading, and or, understanding the conclusion to a logical and truthful explanation. On the contrary, your subconscious mind is more likely to take the opportunity to keep the old program alive. And it will do that by *seeming* to agree with your newfound 'wisdom'.

It could go something like this: You get a strong feeling that suggests that you literally and immediately forget all about your normal responsibilities. If this is your reaction you can be sure that it is not the right course to follow. It is in fact, the old program suggesting action that will not work in order to disprove the new conclusion to which you have arrived. And once your new course of action fails, you then go back to your old ways and declare the new information as false. And the old program remains intact. More than intact, it is strengthened. That's how loyal and powerful your subconscious mind is.

So don't quit your job. We have covered how there is a process involved in changing the constitution of the kingdom - a process that requires time and it requires a process of releasing, and it requires a process of installing the new. The constitution of the kingdom is secure for the very reason that it may serve us well. It serves the purpose of having stability in our lives. Without that stability, we would have chaos. The process of change must be a process within which we can remain secure.

Therefore, let us make full use of our therefore by all means. Let us make use of it to complete our understanding. But let us also be aware that the information we are accepting here has no power in the beginning. New information is just that. It is only information at first. It has no power until it is fully installed. It is information we may well put to good use in time, but it cannot possibly be a part of what we are in terms of having it serve us yet. As has been made clear to us, exposure to new information is much more likely to increase the effectiveness of an older and more established opposite program to start out with.

Once we understand the system and have that understanding fully integrated, we will '*Take therefore no thought for the morrow;.* But before we are fully capable of that, before wisdom would dictate a complete absence of concern for the future, we have work to do. And the start-up to that work is to quit worrying. And that too, of course, has to be a process. It is our excessive, obsessive, and endless concerns that are causing all our problems. It has been made abundantly clear that everything is provided. When we spend all our time trying to create that which is already given, all we do is confuse ourselves, not to mention miss the whole point of what we came here to do. As mentioned, we got so sidetracked with this business of filling our needs that we now spend almost full time with it.

And I know it looks like we need to do that. If we don't get up and go to work, who is going to pay the rent? Good point. And all these things are very real. But the actual problem is that we create these problems just so we can solve them and prove how smart we are. And we do all that because we have this strange notion about ourselves and because we forgot who the real doer of all things is. That's how we keep this merry-go-round going.

But as we start to get back on track with understanding, with acknowledging our source and with working in harmony and with Love for one another, a surprising thing happens. The necessities and even the luxuries of life start to become more easily forthcoming. ***Seek ye first the kingdom of God and his righteousness,*** means just that. It is a process, a process of seeking: it is the process of learning and firmly integrating the ability to use power correctly. And when we get right-use-ness down pat; when we get so that we express righteousness spontaneously, all things are indeed added onto us.

I recently moved into an apartment in a densely populated area where a lot of other old people live. When I first got here I became aware of the sound of sirens very often at all hours of the night and day. I was puzzled by this. I thought that surely there couldn't be that many accidents in a particular area. And then it dawned on me. It was the aged population of the area who were causing all the emergencies. There were frequent heart attacks and the likes to attend to.

But it seems to me that the sounds of sirens at all hours disturbing us is about the last thing we need. The real problem, and what nobody seems to realize, is that the disturbance by the frequent sounds of the sirens is what is *causing* all these heart attacks. So we have a vicious circle going on here that's hard to stop. How do you get out of that one? Do we just let a few of us oldies die to avoid killing off most of the population with the endless sounds of sirens or do we just carry on because we don't know what to do?

Well no, to end a deadlock you have to start by thinking a little differently and make minor changes and these minor changes lead to further changes until we have done a complete turnaround. For example, we might consider using only the warning lights for most of these emergencies. Then we could save the sirens for the really big things like say, an invasion by aliens from another planet. Then by all means play those sirens to your heart's content. But in the meantime, a little peace and quiet might improve our health to the point where even the emergency people might get a little rest once in a while.

Likewise, we have cause and effect backward when it comes to having our needs met. A little concern for real emergencies is appropriate, but we've kind of gone off the deep end here. ***Taking thought for the morrow*** means worry. It's our incessant worrying that is the cause of all our problems. We can get ourselves in enough trouble worrying about today without pushing that forward to the future. ***Sufficient unto the day is the evil thereof.*** We don't need to borrow imaginary problems from tomorrow and add them to the problems we are creating at the moment. That's taking worry to the point of obsession. Worry about the future just nicely keeps us within our self-made limitations, in perpetuity.

So when it comes to our general worries about all the problems in our world that our worries have caused, we can get creative and find ways to cut down and build from that. We can do something like my suggestion of avoiding sirens except for real emergencies when it comes to most of our worries. And just that simple act of freeing our attention to some small degree will give us time to use our imagination to allow further creative ideas to come through. And who knows where that will take us?

Chapter Thirteen

THE BIG TRAP

*Judge not, that ye be not judged.
For with what judgment ye judge,
ye shall be judged:
and with what measure ye mete,
it shall be measured to you again.
And why beholdest thou the mote that is in thy
brother's eye,
but considerest not the beam that is in thine own
eye?
Or how wilt thou say to thy brother,
Let me pull out the mote out of thine eye;
and, behold,
a beam is in thine own eye?
Thou hypocrite,
first cast out the beam out of thine own eye;
and then shalt thou see clearly
to cast out the mote out of thy brother's eye.*

*Give not that which is holy unto the dogs,
neither cast ye your pearls before swine,
lest they trample them under their feet,
and turn again and rend you.*

Looking at the world from the inside of a cab has given me a good bird's eye view of the many follies of what is referred to as human nature. Watching how other people drive can be quite an education. There are any numbers of things I could choose from that are at least amusing if not silly or strange. So, I will choose the simple act of using signal lights because it's my favourite.

If I wanted to be kind, I would say that at least 9 out of 10 people signal incorrectly. But if I drop the kindness and give a more realistic estimate, it's probably closer to 99 out of 100. Do you think I exaggerate? Come for a ride with me and have a look from the high vantage point of a big rig and you will be flabbergasted. And if you look closely, you might even see yourself. Unless you happen to be part of that one percent.

Where do I start? You name it and somebody has done it - all the way to signaling one way and turning the other. Granted I haven't seen that too often, but I just didn't want to leave anything out. I even watched someone signal for every curve on a windy country road one time. I'm not sure what that was all about, but there it was. And then there's signaling too late, too soon, or not at all, or even after the turn is complete. Or the one where somebody has pulled up to a stoplight and then waits patiently until he has someone pulled in behind him and then signals left, making it too late for the person behind to change lanes. And some people do not signal when there is nobody around. The reasoning behind this is that there is no one to signal to. But that reasoning has a flaw or two. One, how can you be sure there is nobody around? How about that short pedestrian behind that tall shrub who was momentarily hidden from your view? Most pedestrians don't signal, but they might need to know where you are going. So if you signal, at least one of you has some information about a possible directional change. And two, what does not signaling when there is nobody around say about habit? You are using your conscious mind needlessly and taking conscious attention away from where it needs to be.

But I'm not finished. My favourite one - and by far the most common - is the fine art of signaling as the person starts to make the turn. All one neat little maneuver. The steering wheel is turned and the signal light is activated in unison. With some people, when they start to turn it's an indication that they are going to signal. And that's not too bad actually. They are on-topic. Signaling is associated with turning. It just needs a little fine-tuning so that it would make sense.

There are others. We really are quite creative. I am often surprised at the inventive way someone has discovered to make the simple act of signaling confusing, in yet another way.

This takes me back to how we do things subconsciously. Of course, we have to do most things entailed in driving subconsciously, but you first have to practice on the conscious level. That means thinking. I may have mentioned that I am in favour of thinking. It can be very useful in learning how to drive. Here is the process: You get the information you need so you will know the right thing to do, and then you consciously and deliberately do these things until they become a habit. After that, you are free to relax and use your conscious mind to watch for all the unexpected variables. Then it's easy. You might even have a bit of spare attention left over to listen to Mozart.

But to get back to the fine art of signaling and turning at the same time, anyone who has adopted that habit is showing promise. He's got the right idea. Signaling does have something to do with turning, but it should precede turning or it sort of defeats the purpose. Close but it does nicely miss the point entirely. What has happened to our star in this show is that he just didn't spend enough time on the conscious level to complete the programming of that which is desired into the subconscious. No big deal and a very common way of doing things. But it does give us a fair view of how some of us run our lives. It's all very understandable. We lead very busy lives and we have a lot to think about all the time. Driving often takes a back seat to other concerns.

I can only assume that all these good people I see who are too busy to signal, or too busy to take time to consider the purpose of signaling, have a life. There's no excuse for me because I have nothing else to do. I should be able to drive without too much effort on a conscious level. At any rate, my driving habits and, or, my inclination towards critical observation, would have me direct at least some of my attention to the study of the strange habits that many other people display.

This is fine and dandy, but it doesn't accomplish anything. Watching other people's mistakes doesn't contribute much to the world or to myself. It makes me a little warier and if I could leave it at that then I have gained something. But my normal tendency as a result of my observation is to be, would you believe, just a little bit judgmental. And that's a deadly trap. If I watch the way people signal and I am simply indulgent of human follies, including my own, then no harm is done. But if I label someone, or if I make an assessment of the people who signal incorrectly, as inadequate, dumb, incompetent, or what have you, then that's a very different thing. With that stance in my mind, I harm myself - big time.

To observe others to categorize, label or judge might seem like a useful activity, and it is certainly the more common thing to do, but it's not harmless and it's not a moral issue. As I have pointed out more than once, there is nothing about morality in anything we are doing here (I just had to flashback to morality there for a moment because it's such a common misunderstanding). As I have explained before, we get nowhere if we include morality into this mix. But *judging* is a trap. You can hurt yourself with judgment. So I need to go back a bit to elaborate. There is an important point here.

The Scribes and Pharisees and the Hypocrites represented the status quo at the time of these biblical writings. And as I have mentioned previously, it's easy now to see how the mainstream mindset at that time needed an overhaul. That was a long time ago, but the Scribes and the Pharisees, and the Hypocrites still exist. They still exist within each of us who are living normal lives. They exist in the good people who are honest, do the right thing, and are the mainstay of civilized society. And they certainly are in full display in my little tirade about the way people signal.

Does that sound a little harsh or hard to believe? Or, heaven forbid, does it sound judgmental on my part? If it does, please forgive me. This is a big issue and I'm still working on it. None of this is meant to be derogatory in any way. I'm just trying to point out a very tricky spot in the process of joining heaven and earth. I'm trying to point out a tricky spot where we God beings get pulled down, down, down, far below anything resembling our natures. The tricky part comes in the form of a subtle trap. It's subtle but it's not small. And I must label it subtle because it's extremely difficult to see ourselves. We have a system set up that doesn't really lend itself to self-reflection. And our world seems to work, so why would we look at it, or look at ourselves, let alone change. But there *is* something wrong. The evidence of that is as close as just a tiny bit of observation. And there is a huge issue here that gets in the way of that introspection.

So here goes:

As I attempt to write this, I see it all at once in my mind. It is difficult to put into words. Difficult because it goes beyond the terms of reference that we commonly use words for. I wish I could just transfer it from my mind to yours without the blemish that words must put on it and complete with Love. Maybe there are those of you who will get what I mean by shutting your mind off and taking that leap to truth. You will just read the biblical quotes and feel the magic, and you've got it. There is something very important here. It can be our emancipation. There is magic in the above biblical quotes so for heaven's sake read that before you start on what I have to say.

You don't have to be schizophrenic to understand this. It's just that it would make it a lot easier for both of us.

But I must assume that there may be normal people reading this so I will use a bit of detail. This is not complicated. It only requires you to turn yourself inside out that's all. But to make this as easy as possible, I will go back to a few basics as reminders so that we can start from that for understanding.

    -We are Divine, great beings capable of all things.
    -The truth about ourselves is not recognized in the world we are in.
    -We live in collective amnesia in terms of this truth about ourselves.
    -That collective amnesia is the mass consciousness and is extremely powerful.
    -Our stance in life is developed at a very early age and is rarely examined.
    -Each child must go through a process of conformity to function in this fictitious world.
    -The biggest problem we have is that we don't know we have a problem.

    Deep down, we know we are perfect Divine beings. That knowing can't be lost no matter how far away we get from reality. That's why I made such a big deal about the extremes we go to, to get attention. As I pointed out then, it's because of that inner knowing that we insist be verified, that we go to so much trouble to get noticed. That attention thing is such a big deal that I was compelled to write three chapters about it. We keep that basic knowing of our perfection and, or, Divinity and take it with us into the fiction that we are presently living. That's why it's so hard to see through the fiction. Yes, we are perfect beings. We just aren't *acting* perfect right now, that's all. And it's that *act* that we have to get rid of before our perfection can come through. But in the meantime, that subconscious awareness of our perfection is so strong that it influences everything we do and how we view the world. And that's the subtle trap.

We come into the world with the knowledge of our true selves and we never fully forget that. We go through a process of conformity in childhood, but our true nature cannot be completely silenced. It stays with us as the background knowing about ourselves because it was our starting point and because it is the truth and because it is way too strong to ever be completely subdued. That knowing has to be a part of us somehow, somewhere, or we would drop dead instantly. It is literally our lifeline. The best we can do is push it to the background. Which is exactly what we do. We push it away until it is only a subconscious knowing. And it's that subconscious knowing that creates the havoc even though it is our greatness. That knowledge of our true selves that we never quite forget is of course a good thing, but it is the trap and the part that does us in. And here's why:

That background knowing is an influence. A very powerful influence and the main motivating force in our lives, even if we don't know it. We keep that or we couldn't function. But it's also this background knowing and feeling about ourselves that defines our entire dilemma. The truth about ourselves is our motivating force and our most powerful influence even though we don't pay conscious attention to it. That powerful, motivating, subconscious and very positive influence is where we get our sense of rightness from. But the outside world and the self we had to create to conform to that world is so demanding that it gets all of our attention. Therefore, *we are each left with our attention focused on the fiction and with living within the fiction but with that sense of rightness about ourselves intact.*

And with a sense of rightness, there is no need for self-examination. Self-examination is subconsciously believed to be dangerous because it could take away that essential image that is crucial for dealing with the world. So we clearly see other people's faults because we see them from that subconscious perspective of our own rightness. We are right about our basic nature, but of course, it's not what we happen to be displaying. But all this is taking place on the subconscious level which is part of the trap because we are unaware of the process in the subconscious by the very definition of subconscious activity.

Now, I know my background presents a fatal flaw in the above hypothesis. But the point of all this is that all people go through a process of conformity and everyone keeps some truth about themselves. So we have a dilemma that we are, quite naturally, unaware of, or it might not be a dilemma.

And here's where it gets crazy.

That sense of ourselves - that subconscious knowing of our true greatness -is not the self we are displaying. So here's the crunch. *The subconscious truth about ourselves is so strong that it overrides awareness of the false identity we must use in order to function in the everyday world.* Only in fiction could such an outrageous thing take place. We allow that subconscious knowing of our greatness into the conscious level because it suits our purpose and because it's about all we have time for. In a harsh subconscious world, you grab at whatever works. In other words, we believe one thing about ourselves but are displaying something else entirely. Yet that false identity is what others see and what we see in others, which leaves each of us with a clear view of everyone else's shortcomings and a blind eye to our own.

So of course we judge one another.

And we judge for another reason too. We also judge because we feel inadequate. Feelings of inferiority and guilt and all the other things that go with living the big lie compels us to want to look better than others so that we can feel better about ourselves. When we take note of someone else's shortcomings, we can rate ourselves as better. We desperately need reassurance in a fictitious world where we have somehow redefined ourselves as less than perfect. So these feelings of limitation we have about ourselves and the natural desire to want to deny them complement the main factor in our compulsion to judge - that left over true knowing about ourselves that I just explained.

So with denial fully ensconced as our way of being, what can we do from the point of view of what is left of the truth about ourselves, but judge? With all this put together, we've got judging down to a fine art. Most of us are extremely good at it.

But of course, this constant and all-pervasive activity of judging or otherwise evaluating and assessing others is not admitted in polite society. If we did that, our world would fall apart. So judging is the unofficial interaction just below the surface. But it is easily observable. We take note of it all the time, even with our humour. Actually, especially with humour because then it's more acceptable. So by all means let's laugh at ourselves. As previously mentioned, when we can start to laugh at our follies, it's a sure sign we are starting to see through it all. And all that is fine except that for our serious and 'meaningful' interaction we do not acknowledge this all-pervasive tendency to judge.

Still, this whole judging thing is not something I would judge as a bad thing. And as I pointed out, we can't call it a moral issue. The fact that we judge each other all the time is not a matter for judgment. It just doesn't work. We can't get to where we are going if we pack that along with us.

I made a big move when I went to a newer computer. That was a traumatic and difficult change for me but I'm getting there. I'm starting to see that it was for the best. I'm getting to like some of the great features my new computer has. And the speed and capacity are truly amazing.

But I had to transfer data from the old to the new computer and that's the part that got my attention the most. That transfer was a one-way street - I was able to transfer to the new computer but I could not transfer back to the old from the new. I had intended at one point to go back to using the old one after having so much difficulty with the new but the old computer could not understand the format of the new one.

And that's what happens to us at a given point on this learning path. Once you have updated your consciousness to a certain point - to the point where you no longer have judgment - there is no going back. Once you have taken that big leap to where judgment is no longer a part of your reality, it renders you incompatible with most of the past. That which represents the past will not be able to accept your new format. And that representation will come in the form of other people. And the ones who are not ready might not be the obvious ones. In a world where things are not always as they seem to be, we can get some surprises as to who is where, and with what.

At this point, not only is it a waste of time, but much harm comes to anyone who tries to give or share his truth with someone who lives exclusively in a physical world. Anyone with whom you may be trying to share your new-found understanding, and who is not there yet, can only take something away from you in order to defend his beliefs. And in that process, something of the spirit is lost to you. And that would be bad enough but the other person is harmed also. That act of defending himself can only strengthen the limiting beliefs. We're on a one-way street with our learning here and there is no way back.

Therefore we need to be discerning in our dealings with others. Some people are so caught up in the fiction that they have lost all concept of their real nature. It is not the better part of wisdom to take these truths into interaction with those who have no beginning of the concept. There is a very distinct line between relinquishing all judgment and discernment. Crossing that line is a common mistake. It's easy to cross that line because as we begin to see the real truth about ourselves, we quite naturally want to share it and we quite naturally see others in a very different light. But some people just aren't ready for this. And we are warned against that pitfall in the strongest terms:

> ***Give not that which is holy unto the dogs,***
> ***neither cast ye your pearls before swine,***
> ***lest they trample them under their feet,***
> ***and turn again and rend you.***

    You have to be able to discriminate; make that distinction. We can hurt ourselves with judgment, but we can also hurt ourselves if we do not use discernment. This is where silence is of paramount importance: Keep everything to yourself, including nonjudgment. There is a certain critical practicality involved here. This is where what we covered about silence and not letting your left hand know what your right hand does comes in strong. Anything you say or do can be used against you by those who are not ready to hear. There is a fundamental rule used in a court of law to that effect and it holds true in all human interaction. Whatever you say can be used against you. No matter what is said, it can be turned around. Anything can be misunderstood and often is in the manner in which we presently interact.

    Nonjudgment starts and ends with silence, which brings discernment. All of which can only be done in and with Love. Love is always silent. How else? How else can we accomplish anything in a world of fiction but stay out of it and hold to Truth? The line between the absence of judgment and discernment can be difficult unless we remember Love. Complete nonjudgment effectively frees Love to flow through, as was pointed out in the chapter on Love. Then we are always inspired to do that which serves our own and everyone else's best interest. The process of reconnecting to Source includes being on the watch for the less desirable characteristics of others, for our protection. This is necessary in a harsh world.

If we can see someone else's limiting behaviour as just that and if we use that information for ourselves to protect ourselves, that's great; but if we identify the person with the behaviour then that falls into the category of judgment. Discernment does not send out judgment. With discernment, you keep the information you have gained, to yourself. And you quietly and calmly go about your business and send out Love and no harm is done.

Where I live, north of the 49th, we wear good protective clothing in the wintertime. We do this out of necessity. It gets a little chilly in the northern climes at certain times of the year. We refer to our winter clothing as warm. We have all kinds of warm clothing to wear; even long underwear and thick wool hats and much more for the extreme cold temperatures.

I have a nice lightweight, down-filled coat that I use on my hikes in my favourite mountain - that mountain where I met my friend the coyote. Well, I'm sure that coyote would not consider me a friend. He made it clear that he doesn't want to so much as associate with me, let alone consider me a friend. But we already established that he is a lot smarter and better equipped for nature than I am in every way. I'm sure his fur coat serves him very well too. It even varies for the seasons.

So given that I am not anywhere as well equipped to be in harmony with nature, I had to remember to put my coat on before leaving for my hikes. Not only that, but I found it necessary to take my coat off partway up the mountain because I would get too warm. But my lightweight coat made it handy to carry up the hill so that I would have it for the way down. I was always very glad to have my coat when my body was generating less heat.

But I noticed something about my coat when I first put it on, after carrying it for about a half-hour or more. It always felt cold. So I learned after a while to put it on just a little before I got to the top of the mountain while my body was still generating that excess heat. That worked well because my body would quickly warm my coat up and then I was able to keep that warmth in for going down.

I concluded that my warm coat contained no warmth of its own at all. My 'warm' coat did not give off warmth, rather it served the purpose of keeping my heat in and limiting the amount of cold that could get through. I have yet to find any warm clothing that actually gives off heat. All of our wonderful warm clothing doesn't really do much unless we have some warmth of our own.

It is the warmth of our Love that protects us against the harsher aspects sometimes displayed in this world. If we do not have Love within us, no amount of protection or security systems can help us. But Love always protects because it is the mighty power and the doer of all things. Love radiates outward and can be used to protect ourselves from any and all that would intrude. Our protective clothing only works if we have some warmth within ourselves and our protection from the coldness we might receive from some who do not understand, is the warmth of our Love as it radiates out. Those who feel and like what you are putting out will respond favourably and those who do not like what you are putting out will feel like being elsewhere.

Everybody feels what you are putting out one way or another. What you are putting out tells a lot about you the same way as it does with the use of signal lights. As in traffic, what we signal to each other in all ways comes from what we hold in our hearts. If we really want to take communication seriously we could start with the signal lights of our vehicles and we could consider this:

Signaling is above all, something you do for somebody else. It is an action we take to notify others of our intent that they may be in an informed position to take necessary action or inaction. It's not something you do for yourself. You already know where you are going, presumably. Therefore, signaling can be considered an act of kindness, even a considerate and loving act. It certainly is not a selfish act. One who signals is considerate of the well-being of others and signals his intent as a contribution to the harmonious flow of traffic.

I wonder what would happen if we all took this concept one step further and adopted the practice of deliberately sending out Love every time we used our signal lights. Soon, signaling would become synonymous with Love. That simple act would probably change the world.

Chapter Fourteen

ASK

*Ask and it shall be given you;
seek, and ye shall find;
knock, and it shall be opened unto you:
For everyone that asketh receiveth;
and he that seeketh findeth;
and to him that knocketh it shall be opened.
Or what man is there of you,
whom if his son ask bread,
will he give him a stone?
Or if he ask a fish,
will he give him a serpent?
If ye then, being evil,
know how to give good gifts unto your children,
how much more shall your Father which is in heaven
give good things to them that ask him?*

I went for a walk with my granddaughter when she was about four years old. As we left the house she seemed concerned about something. I soon found out what it was. We were barely out of earshot from her parents when she turned to me in a very worried and solemn little voice and said, "You know Papa, I can't read."

Imagine such a problem for a four-year-old. Of course, I knew all of the background. I knew that this child had the good fortune of having a mother who read to her every day. And I instantly knew what her real problem was. After being read to since she was a wee baby, she had just now come to realize that words and stories could come from books. She had observed that her mother got the words she spoke by looking at a book. Very impressive observation for one so young. She was fascinated by the concept and quite naturally couldn't imagine that the day would come when she would be able to do the same thing. That was her great concern and very understandable. I felt honoured to be let in on this secret. It was obviously something she didn't dare mention to her parents. I think that this precious child thought she was inadequate somehow. So soon we get indoctrinated into the ways of the world.

But grandchildren instinctively understand that grandparents are different. And the great thing about being a grandparent is that you get your magic back by being with your grandchildren. And when you add that to a little understanding of the ways of the world, it can make for a priceless exchange.

My reply was instant. "You don't have to worry about that. It's easy to learn to read. You already know how to make an A." (I knew she could do this and A is the first letter in her name.)

Her response was a joy to behold. She shouted a happy and exuberant yes and jumped up and down like only a child can do while reaching up and writing an A in the air several times. So simple. A very grave concern solved instantly because of simple trust; trust in expressing that concern.

We have to ask, seek, knock, and above all, trust. There is a higher perspective. There is a higher knowing. There is a higher order of things. There are answers to problems that we can't even imagine. We have capabilities not yet developed that are truly beyond our imagination at this stage. We are like my dear little granddaughter who couldn't imagine that she would ever be able to read. We are indeed like little children in our lack of knowing. But where we differ with little children and to our detriment is in trusting. Every problem has a solution. Every concern, every worry, every fear, needs only a higher perspective that is readily forthcoming for the asking. Who would not give his child the simple necessities of life? Children cannot fend for themselves and need our care until they mature.

Do we really think that all our needs are not provided for? Do we really believe that as children of God, we might not get what we need? Worse, do we really believe that in our apprenticeship, we will not be provided with what we need for learning? How can we not know that we are Loved, cherished, and cared for, much greater than a parent or a grandparent is capable of? No matter how many mistakes and no matter how many times we fall short in any way, the care and Love never varies. But we have to ask. Even if that asking is only expressed as concern, it releases the power of Love into motion: ***For your Father knoweth what things ye have need of, before ye ask him.***

We care and Love and provide for our children in the full knowledge that they can't look after themselves while they are growing up. I gave my granddaughter what she needed in the moment but no more. I didn't try to teach her to how to put a word together. I actually didn't have time to even think about it. She immediately took what I gave her and literally jumped for joy. Now, more than a decade later, she reads and is capable of writing an essay. All that took place in an orderly fashion and in very little time.

What I have learned has been reasonably orderly as well (would you believe reasonably chaotic?). And my first exposure to that which is abstract was quite naturally to the more elementary concepts. I do not know how many stages I've gone through since, but I do know that it is many. There was progression and there still is. I can't begin to know all the background activity that contributed to the ways in which I stumbled on to the right book or the right person or the right situation to encourage and enhance my learning. It certainly wasn't from some formal outline that one might expect in other studies. It's more like I was continually given opportunities despite myself. Still, whatever happened and however it came together and whatever is making it continually unfold, there is no question that I am always given what I need.

And I did indeed ask, even though I did not know what I was asking for at the time. My granddaughter asked indirectly and so did I. And in the same way, I did not know what I needed but something was bothering me. And I couldn't leave it alone even though a solution seemed impossible. I always knew something wasn't right and I spent years reading everything I could get my hands on. I did not know it at the time, but it had to be just a matter of time before my desire for an answer would get results. I had no idea what I was looking for, and not in my wildest imaginations in the early days of my search did I think that I would one day take an interest in matters of the spirit. But looking back now, it was inevitable. It is the only place where the real answers are. Even though I did not know what I was asking for, and my query was anything but direct, I did get answers and I am continuing to get answers. All that is required is an inquiring mind, however vague. That's asking. But if we are complacent about life or otherwise indicate that we are not open to change, that stance is also honoured. Our autonomy makes it imperative that we ask, demand, expect and or otherwise acknowledge our needs one way or another before anything can come about.

Everything is set up and provided for that the learning process may unfold. There is a framework for learning provided. And everything is set up so that we can get on with the business of doing *the greater works* when we are good and ready. But we have to dare to ask. Like my granddaughter did. How could we ever become functional if there wasn't a system in place to give us what we need while we are learning? And even to answer the question of why, when we are ready to ask it. We have free will so that we can do something that has never been done before. God likes surprises. So whatever we need, the supply to make that happen is not the problem. The problem is with us. With us forgetting who we are and imagining that we are these little creatures that live and die and struggle for survival in the interval. That's quite a bit off the mark. We are Beings of the most high with capabilities and a job description that at present seem to be beyond our imagination.

Just one letter of the alphabet was all my granddaughter needed to become confident. What would it take for us adults to get our confidence back? I'm not sure, but we could start by asking, or at least let it be known that we have a concern. Those concerns will be attended to. That's the promise. We have been given quite a bit more than one letter with the information we have here. And now we have come to the reminder that we have to ask. Nothing can happen unless we ask.

The first part of asking is an ongoing inquiring stance as we go along. That's the asking that allows revelation and inspiration to flow. We get just what we need for the moment; just what is appropriate so that we can take the next step. My granddaughter wasn't concerned with trigonometry when she expressed her fear that gaining the ability to read was beyond her imagination. She got exactly what she needed for that moment and she accepted it with exuberant joy.

We have to ask for what we need to suit exactly where we are at; for what we need in the moment and at the level of our understanding in that moment. We can ask, even in fear, and the intelligence vaster than imagination that is built right into our very being, will be activated. All we have to do is work from our point of understanding or misunderstanding. That's the point from which we must ask. We have to ask even if we are confused as to what we want. That simple act brings greater clarity. We have to start somewhere and that somewhere is where we are. We are not judged and we certainly are not measured by the distance we have drifted from reality.

So what is there to add to these biblical quotes? The information we have here is that asking and receiving are one and the same. I don't see a maybe or an if anywhere. It's very explicit. Ask, seek and knock and in every case the answer is in the affirmative. There is no hint of being refused anything. So what's our problem? Aside from the fact that we are often unaware of the contents of our own minds and that those contents contradict what we are asking, what's the holdup? Why don't some, or a lot of us get what we want, some or a lot of the time?

Worthiness! Does that ring a bell with some, or a lot of us? Me thinks it's the big one. Some, or a lot of us do not really have a sense of worthiness which translates to an inability to receive. So there goes asking down the drain. Not much use in asking if we can't receive. But that's why we have been going on and on about a change in identity. That old false identity has to be gently and lovingly laid to rest because it will get in the way. It does not feel worthy of receiving, among other things.

As mentioned many times, our old identity contains a certain sense of separation one way or another. And that sense of separation comes through as a feeling of guilt. And guilt comes from that feeling of separation. We subconsciously feel that there is something wrong with our lack of conscious connection. And that subconscious sense makes us feel as if we have done something wrong. And we are right about that. There is something fundamentally wrong as long as we are not consciously connected to God. But that does not make *us* wrong. Yes, conscious connection is basic to conscious beings by definition but our disconnection does not diminish our basic nature as perfect Divine beings. Our basic nature is not changeable. Our sense of guilt comes from the simple fact that we are not being true to ourselves. That feeling can't be avoided except by those who are extremely obtuse, and or, heavy into drugs or otherwise anaesthetized. The truth about ourselves is a constant and very powerful influence that will not be ignored. But guilt is only a misinterpretation of that truth. Guilt is just the distorted way truth comes through because of the distortion that is our sense of separation. Guilt is not truth. There is no such thing as guilt in higher understanding and guilt only impairs that higher understanding and guilt certainly could never be part of Love. So drop the guilt. All it does is hold things up. We haven't got time for it anymore. We are Loved where we are, with or without conscious connection. The only possible use guilt could have is that we might use it as a motivator to find its real cause.

Which brings out an important point: This whole business of guilt, fear and not feeling worthy of receiving what we want, and or, imagining that we have to elevate ourselves to a certain standard before we can ask for that which would set us free, can be defined in one small phrase: Love for ourselves or the absence thereof. We covered how to get started on the concept of Love in chapter seven, but maybe I forgot to mention that we need to apply that strategy to ourselves. It works.

So we need to get clear on the real meaning of asking. Asking is prayer and prayer is communication. It is communication with cause that we may have the effect we desire. But if that communication has any contradiction or limitation within it, of course that contradiction must be included in the response. Spirit is very exacting and will respond with 100% accuracy every time. Therefore the results from any and all our communication that contains inaccuracies like guilt, unworthiness or any and all other limitations we can dream up, will reflect those inaccuracies.

Everything we have in our minds is asking. Our every desire, our every wish, our every thought is asking. We are asking all the time whether we know it or not. All our thoughts are a connection to cause at all times. That's why it's imperative that we live consciously. That we do not just accept whatever comes into our minds. That we question, ponder and think before we accept whatever pops into our minds. Otherwise we are asking by default.

So if I may answer my own question; the question I posed back a bit? 'What is there to add to these biblical quotes'? Well that was another trick question. Those biblical quotes are way too explicit to leave any room to add to them. The real question is: What is there within our asking that's missing? Or in what way do we ask so that we contradict the request? Or better still: How have we put ourselves in a state where we do not believe that all our needs are there for the asking? How have we managed to get ourselves in a state where we are able to go through a ritual of asking without expecting to receive? And the answer is that we just got a little confused about our identity and that's why we've been a little confused about asking. But our sense of identity is what we have been addressing right from the start. And we know that once we clear all the accumulated debris from our accumulated misunderstanding about ourselves, everything falls into place.

Our power seems to come from outside of ourselves so we have to ask. I say *seems* to come from outside ourselves, because it does indeed come from beyond the self we normally identify ourselves as. The identity most of us have created for ourselves does not include our real self which is always connected to God and is one with God. Therefore, for now, asking is the recognition of that disparity and is the only effective way of connecting to our own power.

But once we get back to expressing our true identity again, our asking will be a command. Asking is effective when it includes the ability to receive. Asking and receiving are indeed synonymous when we speak from the truth of what we are.

THERFORE

Therefore
all things whatsoever ye would that men should do to you,
do ye even so to them:
for this is the law and the prophets.

My circumstances changed and I decided I needed internet. And when I decided to try out email, I thought it would be necessary to send and receive letters as a tryout and that the content would not be valid. It couldn't be valid in terms of exchanging useful or normal information. And then a thought snapped back that I'd be using the system frivolously and that I could get caught. All that took place in a flash and is an example of the absurd thoughts that come into my mind. Of course I discounted all this as fast as it came in, but still, I did have those thoughts as crazy as they were. I didn't say it made sense.

But I couldn't leave it alone. I had to ponder this. Where would such absurdities come from? From some silly subconscious pattern of course. A long way from reality I will grant you, but I have indeed strayed a long way from reality from time to time. But where was I coming from there? What is this pattern, from which these momentary thoughts came, really all about? Well the only explanation I could come up with is that there was, or is, a belief system in existence in my mind that comes from a profound sense of self deprecation. I must have gotten the impression way back sometime that there is an authority that would deny anything that did not fit within a certain strict code, an impression that could only have come from fear and separation. And that childish impression had never been given the light of day until now, so it was still part of me. It was high time to let that go.

Simple reason tells me that the whole internet system runs automatically and that we can all use it as we will.

There is little policing of the net and certainly no monitoring of an old and retired truck driver's email. Who would have the time or even the desire to do such a thing? And who would care about anything as mundane as the information exchanged by email? The whole idea of modern communication is to expedite, not to cause additional work.

So what's frivolous? We are all free to use the internet as we will. Granted there is a lot of garbage on the net, but we may all choose what we want. Even a virus can be avoided with just a little caution and a lot less curiosity. So we're sure not going to overload the system with a few practice runs of email.

And so it is with the way the universe is set up. We're not going to overload infinity while we are practicing and getting the hang of this business of being human. We do not have to ask for clearance of every little detail of our lives. God has already said yes to everything we can imagine or we wouldn't be able to imagine it. Such is the nature of infinity. We have been given our freedom that we might use our God power wisely, or otherwise. And if we choose otherwise, it's just a matter of time until we will see that what we are doing is not working and we will choose again until we figure it all out. We can take forever if we want but it gets a little boring after awhile if we don't try something new.

But we can make it a little easier on ourselves with a bit of understanding. We can spend a little time learning the rules of the game if we want. The truth and the ease with which we may learn are available to us. We can get back to reality anytime we want, which has been the suggestion right from the start with this little endeavour. And we now have a conclusive statement about how it all works:

Therefore
***all things whatsoever ye would that men should do to you,
do ye even so to them:***

for this is the law and the prophets

We've bumped right into the famous golden rule here. Isn't it amazing how some things are so well known? We seem to notice that which has deep meaning and we somehow give it prominence. For sure in my case, I had heard of this long before I ever read one line in the Bible. I think many of us hear these things and it sticks because we subconsciously know that there is a major law of the universe involved. That's how close to the surface our real knowing is. It sure is well named, although it is a little more than a rule. You are indeed going for the gold when you work with this law.

The way I heard it all those years ago was: Do unto others as you would have them do unto you - same thing, just different words. Well not quite the same thing. I had never heard the part about, '*for this is the law and the prophets*'. That changes things a lot. Not that I would have understood that part if I had heard it back then, but it is the part that makes all the difference in understanding. I remember thinking that the golden rule sounded like a very nice thing. Certainly a kind thing and the sort of thing a good person would do. But never in my wildest imaginations did I entertain the idea that this was law, that this was how things actually worked.

We have this conclusion right after that detailed dissertation on asking. We covered asking in the most explicit way possible. So is asking and receiving that simple and that easy? Can we just have whatever we want and do whatever we want just for the asking? Yes. That's how it is. Life is that simple. And life is that good. And there is no but. Unless of course you count universal law and the simple fact that cause and effect can only work in a benevolent way or we would soon blow the place up. Asking has to include our common denominator of course. We have to include Love in everything we do or think or imagine, until we do it in our sleep, literally. So I don't think we can get away with leaving it out of this recipe.

That's how you notify the universe and get the great cause of all things going. That's how to get what you want. That's how you receive - by using the right fuel. The universe doesn't run on high octane or jet fuel or even rocket fuel. Of course we all know what the fuel of the universe is. Therefore to get anything done or get harmony in our lives, we have to employ that which we all have in common. How could anything possibly work if we all did whatever we want to without any consideration for the larger picture? What each of us does affects everyone else or we wouldn't have the power to create.

Therefore ask, seek, and knock by all means. And the 'how to' of that, is simple: Give. Allow Love to free flow through you. That's giving. Giving is as easy as allowing. It's the only way God can know what you want. Since the intelligence of God is deployed only in Love, the software of your intention is compatible with universal intention. The discrepancies pointed out previous to this that get in the way and stop that process, can all be described as an absence of Love. An absence of Love for ourselves as well as what is directed outward. And all our accumulated misunderstanding is represented in the big block which is judgment. Judgment effectively stops the flow of Love because it nullifies our very definition. Judgment is where Love is the least in evidence and that's why we had to get past that before we could get started on understanding the concept of asking.

Therefore there is a little more to this therefore than the conclusion to asking. This is our definitive conclusion involving all previous conclusions. Except for a few important warnings about the pitfalls one can fall into while integrating it all, this is the ending. This is the collective conclusion we may draw from an understanding of everything we have covered right from the beginning.

We started with opening statements that culminated with a clear definition of what we are - that we are *it* in this world as far as creation is concerned: *'The salt of the earth and the light of the world'*. From that we were told that it was time for a complete understanding of ourselves - that this is the final update, ready or not. Then that explanation and the subsequent new definition of ourselves led to the natural conclusion that we are working towards expressing our perfection. And then the common limitations built into our own definition of ourselves were pointed out. And within that, we had clear instructions on how to communicate with cause which effectively redefined us and our purpose: We, as perfect beings, came here to learn to express our perfection in physical forms because there is nothing like tangible expression within which to learn. And we cleared up the most common error about our purpose by learning to ask the right question about ourselves, which led to seeing our priorities in terms of what we might accumulate: The development of our consciousness as a permanent possession over the ever changing things of the physical. And all of this together put us in a position to begin to understand that all our needs are a given. Connecting to Source automatically provides all needs and that we therefore have only to be fully present in the moment to stay out of trouble. Our real challenge has always been to release our self imposed limitations so that our supply may flow freely again as it does in all of nature. From there it is obvious that everything we need is ours for the asking.

So this conclusion isn't just about how to get what you want. What we have here is a declaration of how everything comes about. This is how creation is created. We are, *'Sons of the most high'*. Why weren't we expecting this?

Therefore, with all that background, and now that we have a complete explanation of ourselves and our purpose, we can have another look at the likes of, *'ye are the salt of*

the earth and the light of the world', and get a higher understanding of it. It now becomes obvious that what that really means is that we represent God here on earth. Our real nature is the nature of God / Love. We are now ready to understand the ultimate 'how to'. We are ready to understand how creation works so that we can complete our apprenticeship. We are ready to learn how God creates. This final update is given to us for that purpose. It is indeed time to get on with ***'the greater works'***.

So getting what we want boils down to this: It means going beyond ourselves as we presently know ourselves. And it means recognizing the real cause of all things that cause may be activated. Cause has only to be acknowledged and directed with focused intention to be put into effect. We have to make that conscious connection before we can allow power to flow through us. That's what it means to have autonomy. The great power of God is not ours as individuals, but we do individually express the power of God. And it is by giving that we activate the great power of the universe because creation is a gift. There is no other way to get things in motion. It is the only way we can give notice of what we want to see manifested in our physical world. We, as children of God, have the authority to give and therefore create. And more, all of the above describes our autonomy and therefore our full responsibility for everything in our lives. The nature of God is Love and the nature of Love is to give and that is our nature. Giving is Love in action. This is the great law of the universe: The law of Love that supersedes and contains all other laws within it.

Giving doesn't mean just giving something to someone else. There is a little more to giving than that. Since Love and giving are synonymous, *whatever* you do that includes the well being of others is the real definition of giving. The only way you can have a problem with this is if what you do is exclusively for yourself. It's that exclusivity that gets us into trouble. We are individual, but not separate or exclusive. Defining ourselves as separate is how we cut ourselves from the source of supply and is also why we have to 'work' to get what we want and is also why we are never satisfied with what we have. And that's been our whole problem all along. It's the very thing we are trying to get beyond. So the real meaning of giving, is giving in such a way that it is a contribution to creation. We are creators with God and as God. And with God all of creation is one. There is no separation. The only seeming separation is with us getting so isolated that we forgot our great connection. So as we attempt to fill our needs within that seeming separation, nothing works because there has been no connection to cause. Nobody gains anything in that situation - least of all the one who has so isolated himself. But as we remember our connection and realize that whatever we do affects everything else, we quite naturally include all others in our consideration. And that's giving; that's activating the great power of the universe. *For this is the law and the prophets.*

That's why forgiving works so well. As I pointed out when we were working with the Lord's Prayer, forgiveness is about giving. Miracles take place through forgiveness because you have given notice that you are for-giving; in favour of giving. Once we declare ourselves as for-giving, we connect to, and activate the power. And that giving power, quite naturally, has to run through the one who is doing the giving. And in that process, it has a clearing effect on the misconceptions and limitations accumulated within, and also fulfills all requirements at the same time.

We can't really know ourselves until we understand giving. Once we get a glimpse of our true nature, nothing is ever the same. We look back and are shocked that we could ever have forgotten it. This whole thing spells out how creation works, which of course also spells out how to get what you want.

Let's try it the other way around to help to get rid of any little residual doubt that wants to hang around: What if it was set up so that in order to receive our requirements, we just all take what we want. Sounds easier at first glance but I think we are going to run into a problem. For starters, no one else will know what you are doing, because everybody else will also be thinking only of themselves, which means there would be no communication between any and all of us. So how would we ever get anything done that requires more than one person? But worse, how would we ever make any progress and or expand our sense of self if we lived in a small little world with exclusive self concern? I think that's been tried. It can't work. We are one. And the only way to be functional is to use that basic premise in everything we do. So let's assume that God knows what He is doing and leave it at that and just carry on and do it His way. If God had set it up the way I suggested above, we wouldn't exist because God would not consider anyone but Himself.

How could giving not define our nature since that is the way anything and everything is activated? Not to mention the fact that we are created in God's image. Nothing ever comes into being unless someone activates the potential of infinity by giving. And when we all get that, there will be nobody around to make unreasonable demands. And without unreasonable demands or demands of any kind for that matter, giving will be as natural as the enjoyment of looking at a beautiful landscape. Yes, this does require a little change in direction, but that's what this has been all about and that's why it has been a little challenging once in a while.

I did a bit of golfing for a few years. Among the many skills required is what is called follow-through. I had to think about that. What does it matter what you do after you hit the ball? Surely that's after the fact. It's too late to do anything after you have hit the ball. But no, I came to see that there was an important point here. Of course I'm sure that the mere consideration of anything but follow through is quite laughable to all golfers. But that's okay, go ahead and laugh. Understanding is of paramount importance, even for the most elementary things.

But yes of course, an exuberant and complete swing that actually makes a circle works. It's sort of a celebration of the swing. I remember reading, 'here's to a high finish', as a commentary on follow-through; it is of the utmost importance. Part of the reason follow through is so important is because of what's in your mind as you swing. You know ahead of time whether or not you are going to follow through. And it's that knowing that will greatly affect your swing. Of course any golfer will tell you that it's ridiculous to even consider the necessity of follow through. How could you hit the ball hard and stop there? I never did break 100, but I know that much.

But as crazy as it may be to expect to have success at getting a golf ball to go where you want without follow through, that's more or less what we do if we leave gratitude out of the giving and receiving recipe. Gratitude is follow-through. It works the same way a golf swing does and for the same reason. You know ahead of time what you are going to do. It's about intention and that intention is known to you. And you quite naturally convey that knowing. Without gratitude there is no complete communication with cause and it's about as effective as stopping a golf swing at the location of the ball.

Gratitude, above all, is acknowledgment. Gratitude acknowledges source, and is therefore our connection to power. Gratitude is not just a thank you very much as you would when someone gives you a gift. Gratitude acknowledges our Divinity. Gratitude is the great celebration of what we are.

Follow through is the result of an intention and what we intend is what counts. Our intention is our communication with cause and is received by cause. Follow through and, or gratitude, may seem like it's after the fact but it's not. Gratitude is in the moment of asking because it is already intended and therefore has its effect previous to cause; as it must. Cause must precede effect. God works beyond the limits of time and so do we by our intentions. Our intentions are known just like you can feel what someone's intentions are. Intention is communicated to cause and it is that intention that is put into effect. Intention must acknowledge cause.

When we understand the concept of gratitude and it becomes fully integrated within, it becomes an ongoing built-in part of us and it is our constant connection to cause. We are putting a law into effect by our intentions. The law cannot discriminate and can only work within its own nature. That's the deeper meaning of 'do unto others'. If we withhold Love from anyone or anything, then the law cannot do its work. Loving intention hooks you up with the system.

So to get back to the basics: When we get done with acknowledging and releasing all that makes up our fictitious selves, we can get started on acknowledging our true selves. And as we get back to our true knowing and define ourselves as we really are, we quite naturally and without effort, include everyone and everything in our Love at all times because we finally recognize and feel and know that we are indeed One.

Chapter Fifteen

THE STRAIGHT AND NARROW

*Enter ye in at the strait gate:
For wide is the gate, and broad is the way,
that leadeth to destruction,
and many there be which go in thereat:
Because strait is the gate, and narrow is the way,
which leadeth unto life,
and few there be that find it.*

My granddaughter was the first of the new generation. It was an important occasion when I got that phone call early one morning. I immediately set out to travel from the interior of the province to the coast where my son and daughter-in-law lived. My thoughts were quite naturally filled with this happy event as I made the 4 hour drive and I was determined that this would be a perfect day - that I would not have one negative thought about those with whom I was sharing the highway.

I usually drive as if I'm going somewhere and I have been known to become a little impatient with others who insist on doing just about everything except concentrating on driving. But not this day. I was Mr. loving and tolerance. Well, all except one little incident. I caught up to someone as I often do on a single lane highway. But as I got near, I noticed that we were both going the same speed. That's not the first time this has ever happened to me. It would seem that my presence influenced my fellow traveler. But my reasoning in such a situation has always been that if I caught up to someone, I must have been driving faster than that someone even if it doesn't appear so in the moment. And it's been my experience that if I were to keep following, it's just a matter of time and I would be held up. I therefore take the first opportunity and pass even if the person is varying his speed as was the case this time.

We came to a passing lane and I had to go considerably faster than I had been in order to overtake this person. And soon after that we came to a small town and so I slowed to get at least close to the speed limit. But the vehicle I had passed had been following me and went zipping past me, even though I was going as much as I dared above the speed limit. All this within the boundaries of the town and in an area where passing was not advisable.

Now you can be sure I am no stranger to this kind of behaviour and given the importance of the day, I easily let it go and no harm was done to my emotional state. But I was a little concerned because I knew that the next 50 miles or so was rather crooked and demanded a certain competence that the person had not been displaying. It was most likely that I would experience a delay behind this vehicle.

It didn't take long. I caught up to him going up a hill. The hill happened to have a passing lane and I could have easily passed him again, but I just didn't want to get into that kind of seesaw. And soon we came to another but much longer passing lane on another hill. Of course, I knew this was coming because I had been driving over that road for many years. I know every corner of that road. But what I did not anticipate was that there was construction ahead and that the hill had a long line of cars stopped for a flag person. All dutifully lined up in the right lane.

And then I got a much bigger surprise. My dear antagonist, who had insisted on being in the lead even though he had not displayed any leadership skills, never missed a beat. He didn't as much as slow down. He just took the left lane and went about the business of passing all those parked cars. That wouldn't be so bad, but this story gets stranger. I followed him! I'm still not sure what possessed me to do this, but there it is. That's what I did. I have displayed some rather strange behaviour from time to time, but we better not get bogged down on that subject. I did what I did. But there is yet another strange twist coming up here.

It was obvious that we were both going to look silly stopped where the flag person was standing holding a stop sign. Surely the other lane would be waved on first when the delay was over, and we would just be sitting there looking stupid. But no, that's not what happened. Truth is stranger than fiction, I assure you. Just as we were approaching the stopping area, the flag person turned the stop sign around to where it says slow. The timing was absolutely precise. Our hero, the leader, again did not hesitate and carried on with me right behind him. We had the advantage of just a little momentum so we easily got away before the cars in the other lane could start up.

Now I could tell that this vehicle ahead of me had considerably less power than my big V8, and I knew we had plenty of passing lane left and I also realized that there would probably be no traffic to catch up to, given the obvious long delay that had just ended. And I also knew that there were no more passing lanes for many miles. I am sure I don't have to tell you what I did. I gave it a big burst and not only smoked the guy at about double his speed, but I never saw him again. As I expected, there was no contest when it came to serious driving, and I had the road to myself. A real breakaway.

So, all is well and I have a space to myself with nobody else around and I carried on in happy anticipation of meeting my new granddaughter. Well for a little while anyway.

I did enjoy my freedom for the remainder of that twisty part of that road and all the way to where we come to the freeway and to a big sign in the middle of the road directing all traffic to a police vehicle check. No big deal, my car was fine even if a little old. I was confident that it would pass. But it didn't. A kindly policeman noticed a small crack on the very bottom corner of my windshield. It was in no way an obstruction to my vision. You would have to go out of your way to notice it, but this wasn't good enough for the one in authority. I was given a ticket. Only a work order to replace the windshield actually, but this did not please me. My car was big and old, with a one-piece windshield and I was a little hard up and none of this made sense. It was going to cost me almost the worth of the car to replace a windshield that did not need replacing at all. Nothing about this episode came even close to making sense.

Unless of course, the universe was keeping track of all activities and using this opportunity to affect a balance from my escapade with that incompetent driver back there somewhere. Not to mention many people in that line up who may have seen my behaviour as rude.

But that's not counting my real concern. This was the day that must not be marred under any circumstances. But it was. And I knew there was no way out of it. I had this ticket in my pocket and I knew that these things are all recorded on a computer and there was nothing to do but obey and pay. And worse it would always be a record in my mind on this day. It was just too much to handle so I just refused to think about it and carried on to my destination. Without further incident by the way.

I actually allowed myself to forget about it and concentrated on my purpose. My son was delighted to see me and couldn't wait to take me to the hospital to show me his beautiful new daughter. It was a happy occasion. I stayed overnight and we had a fine celebration.

I left the next morning. During the drive, I had time to review the events of the past day. And there it was. There was no escaping it. That special day had been blemished. But I just couldn't tolerate it. So, I did me some very serious communicating with God and let him know that this was more than I could bear. And it wasn't long before I sort of felt okay with it, even though I couldn't explain why. And at about that same time I was coming up to a fork in the road where I could continue the highway I was on or take an alternate route. The road I was on was by far the best, but it had a long steep hill on it that caused me a little concern for my old car. I was afraid it might heat up. And I had also been having a little trouble with the battery, so I did not have my lights on, even though this was and is something I am strict about. I use my lights no matter what the conditions are. Anyway, given the condition of my car, I decided to take the alternate route to avoid the big hill. And just as I turned on to the other road, it occurred to me that I should use my lights because this was a two-way road whereas the one I was leaving was a freeway. I was not quite as concerned about lighting on a freeway. But then I thought, no, it will be all right, the hell with the lights. And then bang! It was like someone yelling at me. It came into my mind so strong that I had to obey. PUT YOUR LIGHTS ON!! So, I did. And I got about 2 miles down the road to another surprise. Wall to wall red and blue again. Another police check.

      I wasn't too worried even if I was surprised to find this on an old country road. I had just gone through a check and I knew it couldn't get worse. But now that I think about it, where do we get that expression, 'things can't get any worse'? Maybe we should be careful with such statements. I rolled my window down as I pulled up to the policeman who waved me over. Without so much as a hello, how are you, he said, 'put your high beams on'. That wasn't too hard to do. I complied and he promptly informed that I had a headlight out. That would be okay, but he didn't leave it at that. Again, with no discussion he wrote me out a ticket. This was truly a man of few words. I was so shocked; I was literally speechless. I just crumpled the ticket up and stuffed it into my shirt pocket.

What's going on here God? I asked for a little help. Just a small miracle is all I asked for because I simply do not have the capacity to tolerate the results of the events of yesterday. Instead, things get worse.

I got as far as just around the first corner, which was no more than 100 yards away, when the light went on. No, no, I don't mean the headlight. The proverbial light inside my head. This is the 7th today. Yesterday was the 6th. If I change the headlight and take my ticket to any police station, the record will show my car clear! I got my miracle! I just didn't recognize it right away. Good thing or I would never have been able to hold still while I was getting this second ticket. Thank God for computers and the simple fact that they can't think. Once the computer gives my car a clean bill of health on the 7th, well of course it couldn't show anything wrong previously. So, I stopped on the way home and happily picked up a headlight and installed it. And then I promptly went to a police station and brought my ticket in. That policeman didn't even check. He just asked if I had replaced the headlight and took my word for it. This is not the kind of thing that causes grave concern to the police, me thinks.

Five years later, I sold that car for 100 dollars. And it still had the same windshield. The 6th was indeed a perfect day and we celebrate this story every year on this day. Can God work retroactively when necessary? Of course!

And me? Well, I'm still working on being more tolerant of those with whom I share the highway and I'm making a little progress. That episode helped a lot.

I asked. I asked with a quiet determination because my back was up against the wall. And I asked not just for myself. I asked out of Love. And from Love, my own follies were canceled so that Love could do its work. This is the most beautiful story I know. There is a law that supersedes all other laws including our man-made laws.

I've told this story many times because it's a great story and it's a success story. It's the success of successes. What more is there than making a connection and receiving a miracle? But I also tell it for another reason. I always enjoy telling this story because I feel so good about it. I feel that I really pulled one off there. Hard to top that story. In other words, I brag about it.

But now, these many years later, I see that this bragging motive kind of misses the point. As I review this story carefully, I must ask myself what there is to brag about. What did I do that was so wonderful? Yes, it is a huge success story. No doubt about it. And it certainly has a happy ending. And all these things are good. But maybe I should take another look at my part in it - all the details. Isn't this what I am always advocating: That without real honest introspection, we cannot make any progress whatsoever.

I think I missed that straight gate there. It's a lot narrower than I thought. I did miss it. I took the broad way because it was much more obvious. More than obvious it was extremely enticing. I lapped this all up with great relish because it made me look good. It's only now that I can see that my interpretation of it was all about me. I fell into this whole thing about 'to be seen'. There was sure nothing secretive about 'my' accomplishments. My right hand knew fully well what my left hand did, and so did everybody else around me. I did not take heed like I might have, had I known and taken to heart the admonishments we covered so thoroughly in chapters 8, 9, and 10.

To start with, I sort of missed my first cue. When I caught up with my fellow traveler with whom I had the difficulty, I could have made a different choice than I did. I could have just stayed behind him. He had clearly shown me his colours. Any engagement was going to be trouble. I could have considered that and acted accordingly. As I pointed out earlier, I've been there many times. I know better. I know that nothing good can come from such a situation unless I turn the other cheek. ***Go with him twain*** indeed. Ideally, I could have concluded that I was dealing with an obstruction. Sometimes there are delays on the road for any number of reasons. Who would know that better than me? And there have been times when I have made a different choice and the result has always been good. There have been times in similar situations when I totally accepted the situation and the person. And always, always, I have received my freedom from such a stance. Either the person pulls off the road or turns off or something happens where I don't have to do anything, and the situation is resolved. I know better and I could have made a different choice but I did not and the situation escalated. ***Agree with thine adversary quickly.***

And then I had another chance when he passed me driving like a maniac through that small town. That was a pretty big clue. Something was amiss here. I had engaged someone who was clearly in a dangerous state of mind. And I got that. I stayed behind when I could have passed him again. But something came over me when he pulled that stunt of passing all those stopped cars. I guess I wasn't at peace with this as much as I let myself believe. I followed him like a blind man. I followed him physically just like I had been mentally and emotionally. And look what I did after he and I have the unbelievably good fortune of not paying the consequences of this outrageous act, but instead we are set free to carry on. There certainly was no stopping me then. Of course, I took the opportunity to be rid of him once and for all. Especially considering that I knew full well that I would have the road to myself after that. There was no question about my choice at that point.

I believed I had it made there. All seemed to have taken place in fairness and I carried on in full confidence that I was fulfilling my mission of having an unblemished day. After all, I had exercised some restraint around this situation.

It seemed that my breakaway was my due. Until the roadblock that is. That was a rather rude awakening, and I got the connection.

I understood the whole process on the way back. I asked for help the next day in full awareness of the chain of events and fully cognizant of the cause and effect involved. I had a change in heart. And I followed the prompts after that even if I did have to be hit over the head to get my headlights on. If I hadn't had my headlights on, I'm sure that cop wouldn't have asked me to put my high beams on. He must have been hard pressed to find something wrong. Little did he know that he was doing God's work. At least I assume he did not know. Still, he was a man of few words, so there is no telling where he was at.

I didn't understand the nature of the process that was going on there immediately either. That had to be the biggest shock of all when that sunk in. Miracles are something like accidents. They always come as a big surprise in this state of disconnection from Source in which we are presently having our experience.

So, bragging about this episode leaves some rather important factors out. Like the fact that I created a series of negative circumstances that normally would have cost me big time. Or that I was released from my own folly by the Grace of God. Or the strong possibility that God takes great care that only the best circumstances exist surrounding the entry of one of his children into this world. Yes, I wanted only good on the day of my granddaughter's birth, but I think God was way ahead of me. It's more like God took care of everything despite all the destruction I seemed bent on causing.

But even with all that, I did do something right, though I didn't know it at the time. I set a clear intention. I wasn't wishy-washy about what I wanted. I asked. I definitely asked. I asked and I received. Normally, I would not have had that capability to receive, but I was desperate.

Desperate enough to let it go because I knew there was nothing I could do. I gave it up because I had to, and that's what let the miracle come through.

I messed everything up after my original intention of having a good day and got myself into nothing but trouble and the only way out was to do nothing. But I did ask. That's the real meaning of asking and that's why we use the word, ask. It acknowledges the real doer of all things. Left to my own doing it's obvious that I would have left a trail of disaster behind me. But I asked and it was given me. *If ye then, being evil, know how to give good gifts unto your children, how much more shall your Father which is in heaven give good things to them that ask him?*

That's the straight gate; that's the narrow way. And it's narrow and not obvious because it's not where we spend most of our time. The world as it is, is glaring in its influence. It's not that easy to ignore all the normal ways of seeing things and doing things. At least it hasn't been for me.

And that's why we have this warning here. The draw and the influence of the ways of the world that would stop us from awakening to our true selves, is subtle and strong.

Chapter Sixteen

BEWARE
(oh wow)

*Beware of false prophets,
which come to you in sheep's clothing,
but inwardly they are ravening wolves.
Ye shall know them by their fruits.
Do men gather grapes of thorns, or figs of thistles?
Even so every good tree bringeth forth good fruit;
but a corrupt tree bringeth forth evil fruit.
A good tree cannot bring forth evil fruit,
neither can a corrupt tree bring forth good fruit.
Every tree that bringeth not forth good fruit
is hewn down, and cast into the fire.
Wherefore by their fruits ye shall know them.*

My oldest grandson and I made plans to go for a walk on a certain day when he was in his fourteenth year. But when I arrived at his place at the appointed time, he had changed his mind. He professed great fatigue. Well, I suppose that could have been true. Who knows what the pressures of school and life are for a teen these days? But I was quite sure that what he was really suffering from was inertia. The way he was stretched out on the couch was my big clue. Not to mention the insidious and debilitating influence of daytime television. So, I just wouldn't put up with it. I insisted that we carry on as planned. I also assured him that I could call 911 on my cell if he should collapse on the way. He finally got tired of my coercive ways and acquiesced.

And it wasn't long after we started walking before his mood changed considerably. And more, he soon took on an entirely different persona. He became very jovial and fun to be with, his usual self. He even expressed his pleasure that I had insisted on the walk.

So on the way home in the car, we somehow got on the topic of the great difference on how he now felt compared to how he felt earlier. He seemed surprised that he could undergo such a change. I explained to him, along with the usual rider that that was what grandfathers are for and how lucky he was to have such a good grandfather.

Pretty elementary stuff in my explanation, but some of these things seem to get lost in our modern-day lifestyles. Indeed, we could probably make better use of our elders if we could possibly squeeze them into our busy lives.

But anyway, this moment was presented to me and I delighted in the opportunity. I explained to him in simple terms that our bodies, when in a state of rest, are inclined to stay that way unless we take action. We must take command of our bodies and when we do, our bodies respond surprisingly well. I explained further that what he had done was let his body control him rather than take control of his body. When we have things in the right order, with the mind in command of the body, everything works as it should. That's the way it's supposed to be. But when we let our bodies dictate our actions, we cannot possibly expect good results. The body does not have the ability to make the big decisions. Yet, it does make decisions to keep it in optimal running order all the time - like healing for example. But it does not have the ability to decide on its own direction; it can only obey direction. And it does that very well. It will do its best to continue to rest for example, if that's the command it has received, even if that command was by default.

And then I went on to declare that taking command of our bodies really means taking command of our minds. That got his attention. He said, "I thought I was my mind."

To which I quickly responded, "No, you are not your mind or how would you be able to change it."

But I was very pleased that he had his brain in gear. He must have thought about this at some time. He was actually making good use of his mind without realizing it and showing great promise. Very gratifying in a world of pre-cooked thinking. A great joy to be able to have such an exchange.

His next question came very quickly. "Well, what am I then?"

He thought he had me there. This was truly one of those moments that you can't make up. It just has to happen when it's time and I was fully aware of it. I had to watch myself not to laugh at his tone of voice which suggested there could not be an answer to this. All this took place very quickly and my response was at least at the speed of light.

I said, "You're a spirit!"

Big silence. End of topic.

I did not take it any further. That was enough for the day. There may come a day when he has further questions. Who knows, he might even ask me what the purpose of life is someday. And I will tell him that by a happy coincidence I just happen to have written a book on that topic and that the purpose of life is to be and that it is the only real question we are ever faced with. We must all choose to be or not to be, the same as we must all choose to get up off the couch and go for a walk. Or not. Or I might just take off where we left off. I could say, "Now that you know that you are a spirit, the next big thing you need to know is that we are here to learn to choose."

As a spirit, you already are perfect so the whole trick to life is to learn to make the right choices so that you can eventually learn to express that perfection in this physical dimension that we call earth. And that's the real meaning of 'as it is in heaven.' We needed a name for what we can't see and where our perfection already is, so we called that heaven. And then I might go on to explain that the way the world is set up right now, we must work at it a bit to get back to expressing what we really are. But don't worry, that's what we are here for and there are plenty of ways of getting back on track. What is important though, I would explain, is to realize that something is wrong and to therefore look at other possible ways of doing things and to question everything and see if it seems right to you. Because by far the most predominant influence around us would have us keep things as they are. The easy way is to just go along. But that's wasting your life. That would be like letting your body decide not to go for a walk.

And then who knows, when he gets older, in the next installment I might tell him that we are the thinking part of infinity. That it is only through thinking that anything ever gets done in the universe. And that that's our whole purpose. Conscious, deliberate, directed thought, is how the intelligence and the potential of the universe are activated. And so of course, that can only be done by conscious beings. If it wasn't for conscious beings, infinity would just be static possibilities. Only conscious beings can decide to be what they want and create what they want which means directing infinity as they will. I would inform him that without exercising our right to free will, we technically are not being. That we give up our nature which is to be. Without exercising our free will, we are choosing by default and we are not choosing to be. And that's why every question about ourselves boils down to: To be or not to be?

And I would also warn him that his mind will take him all over the place if he lets it, just like it did by insisting that he stay on the couch. Your mind will take you here and there as if it could change the past and manage the future. But of course, it does not have any power at all, let alone that kind of power. That kind of power is reserved for *You*. The main function of the mind is to manage the present. Therefore, it is completely derelict in its duties if it is anywhere else. It's like not showing up for work. *You* can think whatever you want. *You* can direct your attention and your thoughts as you wish. *You* can effectively structure your thoughts as *you* will. Therefore, *you* are not your thoughts or even your mind that entertains thoughts. Your mind and your thoughts are at your command. And since *you* have the power and ability to take command of your mind and thoughts, your mind is not who *you* are.

I would point all this out, even though it is self-evident, for a good reason. Many of us act as if we are our minds. We let our minds take control to the extent of forgetting the simple fact that we have the control.

Your mind is the manager of your affairs. But it must take orders from the chairman of the board, which is *you*. If you allow your manager total freedom it can take you here and there and everywhere, and to what may not be in your own best interest. The manager is just that; a manager delegated to keep things orderly and keep things running smoothly, but it cannot and does not have the ability to make the decisions about the direction the company wishes to take. The manager must take orders from the owner of the company. What all that means is that the owner of the company is the one to take a new direction or change with the times or institute different policies. You have complete autonomy, and **You** are not what you think. And yes, that has a double meaning.

Yes, I would say all that. What greater privilege and joy could I have than to explain life to my grandchildren?

***

I look out my window and I notice a great movement in the trees. This is caused by the wind. If it wasn't for the wind, those trees would never move. Well, maybe when a bird lands on a branch or something like that. But the movement of a tree must come from an outside force. The trees do not have the capability to move on their own. No doubt they enjoy the movement caused by the wind, but they can't make that happen. Their capabilities keep them quite limited. They are even limited to one location for a lifetime. Plants are very limited, even though there is variation in how they react to the environment. Animals are not nearly as limited, but their choices are limited to their instinct. But even at that, there is much variation in choices. Each animal has its own unique character.

But when it comes to us, any comparison to other life forms can't really be done. Our choices are not limited, and we are not limited. We can think. We can think and make decisions and then think some more and try again and choose again and build on to that indefinitely. Our freedom is absolute. And our choices are literally infinite. We can move or remain inert. It's all a matter of choice. We can choose what we do with our bodies. In fact, we have to choose or nothing ever gets done and we never get anywhere or get what we want. And if we make a mistake, we can simply choose again. We can make mistakes and take note that that's not really what we wanted and then make another choice. No matter what choice we make, it's changeable. The results of a past choice may not be changeable but we can always make new choices. Complete freedom of choice is what defines us from all other life forms to the extent that any comparison can only be limiting. We are only limited by the limitations we impose upon ourselves - by how we define ourselves.

But that has to be a two-way street. Our freedom means we can and do choose whether or not we will get out of bed in the morning, or off the couch in the afternoon. And we choose what we think we are. And we can make mistakes in both cases. We can try vegging out all day on the couch and then decide that we didn't like the results and choose again the next day. And we can define ourselves as the bodies we occupy and then entertain other possibilities until we come to a greater understanding of ourselves. We can ponder and work at figuring out our own nature until we know ourselves completely. We can know ourselves as completely autonomous, conscious beings through the ability we *have* as completely autonomous, conscious beings.

We can even investigate the innermost working of our minds and our emotions and feelings and learn how to use all that information to our best advantage. And in that whole process, in that investigation, we will come up against what we are not. We will quite naturally notice any and all errors in understanding about ourselves that we may have made in the past. Then it's just a matter of time and we will see that we are not our bodies or our minds, or even our feelings.

But we are getting a little closer to the truth about ourselves when we start investigating our feelings. Now we're getting somewhere. If we need one word that would describe what we are, and if the word spirit is too vague, then we have a better word that comes complete with feeling. There is a word that is a little easier to relate to and to which we have some experience and certainly feels good, and that word is Love. So, the day will come when we know ourselves better and we will make a truthful declaration about ourselves by saying, "I am Love. Love is what I am. Love is my nature. I was conceived and created in Love. The creator has no other material with which to create. How then, could I be anything but Love?"

And that's the simple truth of course, but that's jumping ahead a little. As truthful as that statement is, it would be a mistake to try and make that leap without the understanding that leads to that conclusion. And that understanding comes about by clearing and releasing any and all of the false identities we have taken on - the imposters that have taken the place of Love to such an extent that we have forgotten what we are.

It is indeed only through our feelings that we can really answer that big question: 'What am I?' How else but through our feeling could we become aware of God and therefore of our own nature? None of our normal five senses are going to inform us of God's presence.

So, the obvious conclusion is that we have to get clear on feelings. We need to get tuned into our own feelings. We have no tangible evidence of God or what we really are so I don't see how we can get around this. Feelings are the key. What could possibly be the problem? How can we be unaware of God and the truth about ourselves would be a better question? We must have the ability to be aware of our connection or how could we ever get on about doing what we are to do. It's obvious that we are hardwired for that connection, so I'm going to start with that basic premise and see where it takes me.

The next conclusion is obvious. Since we are hardwired for a connection, there must be a problem with the connection. Therefore, there must be a problem with our feelings. We are not *feeling* connected, or we wouldn't have any problems. It has been made abundantly clear that once we are properly connected, everything we could possibly need is always forthcoming and everything works in harmony. We certainly have covered that thoroughly. And since we already know what the only possible connection can be, our problem must be something to do with that connection, with our feelings. So, what is there to do but take a good hard look at our feelings?

I'm going to start by breaking it down a little. According to my dictionary, there is some difference between the definition of feeling and emotion. Emotion describes our more reactionary feelings like fear and the likes, whereas the word feeling is reserved for that which could be termed more sensitive and without the reaction. So maybe we're onto something here. There was no shortage of fear around the last time I checked. Let's have a look at that and see if that helps. I will investigate fear and at least some of its derivatives and see where that takes us. I've had a few experiences with fear and one, in particular, that helped me to understand it firsthand.

***

On nice days when I had the time and the inclination, I used to extend my hikes up my favourite mountain to part way up the next range. And on one of these excursions, I had a nice surprise. Something caught my attention in my peripheral vision. There were two of the cutest little baby bears playing, less than 100 yards from me. They were so tiny that it was obvious they were of that year (Baby bears stay with their mother into the second year). They were having such a good time, and I was so enthralled by the performance, that I just stood there a while watching them. But for some reason something else popped into my mind. I had the thought that where there are baby bears, there is a pretty good chance there is a mama bear. I slowly turned my head to scan the area and I didn't have to look far. There she was, no further from me than the baby bears, just over a bit. Not only watching intently, but I had the distinct impression that she had been watching me the whole time I had been watching her babies.

So, I abruptly lost interest in this little sideshow. I had the presence of mind to look straight ahead and slowly resume my walk, trying to act very casually about it. But I don't think my movements looked very natural. At least I felt very stiff, but I just concentrated on getting out of there and not looking back. That worked. Or at least nothing happened. I never heard a sound, but I had the strong feeling that mama bear's head was slowly turning to keep track of my departure.

After a mile or so I started to relax. She had not come after me. I had it made. I had heard stories about how fierce a mother bear can be when it comes to her young, so I was very relieved. I still had to get back home, but there was no way I was going back that way. I would do whatever it took to find another route. I knew that if I kept going far enough, I would eventually get to a highway. Although this was way out of my way and I would have to hitchhike home, it would be well worth it.

But as I relaxed more, I got to thinking of a better way. I knew the area well and I reasoned that if I took a long route home but over a ways, I would be okay. So, I started back on a path a good distance from where I had been and eventually came to a big clearing that I usually avoid. I knew at that point that I was adjacent to where I had seen the bears but I was at least a half-mile away so I felt confident that I was out of mama bear's range. Big mistake. Apparently, bears have a bigger range of hearing or smell or whatever than I knew about. I heard a crashing sound like something running through the woods. I thought, 'no, it couldn't be', knowing full well that it was. I looked over to where the sound was coming from, and soon there was that big snout coming into the clearing. Mama bear and I must have had a little misunderstanding. Or at least there was a gap in my understanding.

That's when I found out how fast I could run. I knew that I wasn't going to get a second chance at a slow departure. I remember the sound of the wind going by my ears. I really surprised myself at my own speed. That doesn't mean that I could have won the race, but with my little head start, mama bear and I got far enough away from her babies that she changed her mind. Or maybe she decided she had achieved her purpose. I don't know. All I know is that she must have stopped and turned around because when I eventually dared to look back, she was gone.

I also remember cursing my own stupidity for not listening to myself earlier when I had decided to go to the highway.

I know a little more about bears now and I did learn something from that coyote I mentioned way back when. But there must be an easier way to learn about nature and I hope there is an easier way to learn about our own nature. Maybe I should just stick to the city as long as I am compelled to daydream when I'm in the woods.

But I did learn something about fear.

***

That was my research into fear, but I must admit that it was definitely not planned. The purpose of fear is to release adrenalin so that you can run faster if a bear is chasing you. Fear can come in real handy sometimes and it's built into our makeup for a reason. Fear is definitely an e-motion. It certainly got me in motion.

Fear was meant to work as a temporary boost to get all your faculties going as high as they will go. And it's worth it if it saves your life but it does take a toll on the body to be running on full alert and full power. If this high alert is kept on too long or even if we operate on low alert on an ongoing basis, it's going to have the opposite effect than that of saving your life. It must. It was never meant to be our day-to-day motivator. Everybody knows that using adrenaline taxes your body big time.

So, we got a little carried away when we let fear be part of our everyday thinking. Especially when you consider that there are hardly any bears in and around the city. Fear has its place, but we have incorporated it into the very fabric of how we do things, into our motivation for ordinary activities. We got too involved with fear because of our sense of separation. As long as we have a sense of separation from Source, we are going to have fear. That's how fear got so exaggerated. Fear kicks in when something is wrong, for emergencies. *But life is not an emergency!*

The constant use of fear - even in small amounts - is a natural part of our unnatural world. We use fear just to get our day going. We use the word alarm for the device we have to stop our rest and forcibly get going in the morning. We live by the clock, and we start our days by having our clocks alarm us. That wouldn't be so bad, but we consider that normal. So, we've got a problem here. When we have taken this separation thing to the point of scaring ourselves to get started in the morning just to make sure we have fear in place, we've gone too far.

Let's visit Mama Bear again. Let's take another look at that basic emotion that we got a little too carried away with and run a little comparison with what could have been. Mama bear gave me an experience with fear in its pure form. But what could I have done differently? If I had been a little more identified with my real self, what choice would I have made?

When the episode began, I had no fear whatsoever. When I came across the little bears playing, I simply enjoyed their presence and was quite enthralled with watching their play; it was simple and innocent. But then that thought of Mama bear came into my mind. I think her presence and her focus on me finally got through and that's what caused me to consider her. And when I saw her, everything changed. Fear kicked in just like it was supposed to, and I took the appropriate steps, literally - although those steps were a little stiff. But even with the predominance of fear, I knew enough to go easy and make my departure as quietly and as dignified as possible. That knowing came from my spirit. Even though fear was doing its work as it was meant to, I also knew enough not to let fear dictate my actions completely. I did have the presence of mind to control that fear. My fear served me, but I could not afford to have it overwhelm me. And that worked. It got me out of there.

There I was. No harm done and it was a very interesting experience, complete with high drama. The wisdom of my spirit had dictated my actions and I came away unscathed. I was very clear on what steps to take to avoid further danger. But no, after a while, I made a different decision that seemed perfectly reasonable to me. That didn't work so well. And I was extremely lucky to get out of that one. Although my fear served me well again, it was much more extreme that second time.

But what happened there? The problem was solved. What caused me to change my mind and make a very poor decision? What started this process of reasoning? How did I get a new idea and a new game plan going? Those are tough questions to answer. I was so puzzled by my behaviour that I played it back to myself later.

It must have started with a feeling. It had to. Feeling is our great connector and precedes the reasoning process. The job of reason is to check and see if our feelings are worth acting on. That's how we keep our inner balance. If we just acted on every feeling without reason, we could get into big trouble. That's the checks and balances that are meant to keep us at optimum operating level. And in this case, my reason found a reason to agree with the feeling, which I subsequently acted on it.

What feeling started that process that served me badly? That's the real question. Can we not trust such a feeling? Is that what that means? No, it does not mean that we cannot trust our feelings. But it does mean that we must examine our feelings to see if the program they come from makes sense. This is what we must do in the state we are in because feelings may very well come from some erroneous belief system - as long as we have an erroneous way of living our lives. And I will explain how our feelings can keep us stuck, shortly.

But first, here's what happened to me as a result of obeying my feelings to the point of letting it override common sense: That feeling was so insistent that I let it affect my reasoning to my detriment. And that's why we must understand our feelings better. A lot better. I got in touch with my real self in that first emergency only because that situation was beyond the abilities of the self I normally identify with. I didn't know what to do when I first saw mama bear and my need for survival was so extreme that my higher knowing kicked in. In other words, I exceeded my normal boundaries. My spirit took over and gave me information that handled the situation perfectly, but only because my normal knowing shut down and because it did not have the capacity to handle the situation.

That's what caused the problem and caused the backlash.

My 'normal' self was very threatened by having its inability revealed and had to take steps to regain its position of authority at the first opportunity. And so, my feelings about the situation came up and reason helped out and suggested an 'easier' way to get home. 'I', that false me, took back control. That counterfeit self - based in fiction - cannot afford to have an authority claim superiority over it or it will be exposed and that would spell its demise. So 'I' made a very bad decision so that 'I' could survive. But ironically that survival decision almost caused the opposite. How's that for a false prophet? Giving out false information to the point of being suicidal. That's how steeped in fiction the false self is. That self is an illusion, but it has taken on a life of its own as if it was real and therefore will take whatever steps necessary to keep that illusion alive to the point of self-destruction and still not see the error. It cannot see the error because it – it, itself, *is* the error.

That's the basic flaw in how we operate and how we keep that same basic flaw going in perpetuity. This basic flaw in the system, and in the way we keep our fictitious self alive, is what keeps us away from spirit and from our own real knowing and from the harmony of the universe. And yes, it's all about fear, but that doesn't mean we should be fearful about it.

My encounter with mama bear gave us a clear picture of fear in all its glory. Fully capable of serving us in an emergency just like it is designed to do, but so inadequate for the normal decisions of life that it actually works in reverse. It does the opposite to serving us. Rather it keeps us stuck right where we are with no chance whatsoever of getting hooked up to our spirit again.

> *Beware of false prophets,*
> *which come to you in sheep's clothing,*
> *but inwardly they are ravening wolves.*

So that's our real false prophet. And it does indeed come in sheep's clothing, and it is indeed a ravening wolf that would devour us. Our false prophet within is represented by all emotion that has its base in fear.

So, let's go all the way back to where we started investigating our feelings. We have exposed the problem: Our secondary feelings, more commonly referred to as our emotions, most often override our true feelings because we have set it up that way. Let's get right at our emotions and see what can be done about them because they're getting in the way.

To start with, our emotions are after the fact, so we don't want to mess with our emotions directly. At least we don't want to try to subdue, repress, or otherwise try to get rid of our emotions. Emotions as after the fact mean that the function of our emotions is to report what's happening within us, among other things. The last thing we want to do is ignore our emotions. Our emotions are the truth about where we are at. Even if that truth is not what we really want. For example, we might feel resentful or jealous. Even though we might wish we did not have these feelings, they are the reality of our lives in the moment. It is essential that we acknowledge our emotions before we can make any kind of a start at understanding ourselves and go from there.

There is a critical point here: We do not ignore our emotions under any circumstances; anything but. That's extremely dangerous. We must never, never do that. As I mentioned in chapter three, that's the kind of thing that leads to Mr. nice guy coming to work and shooting all his co-workers one day, seemingly for no reason whatever. He has suppressed his anger and it built up over time to the point that it finally took on a life of its own and it overcame him, and it had to be expressed. We absolutely must be aware and acknowledge and find some way to express our negative emotions as we go along. We must not ever ignore our emotions. They are indeed the powerhouse of our makeup in the state we are in. We have had enough examples of what happens when emotions get completely out of control. Above all we must acknowledge our emotions before we can even think about understanding them and making changes. Acknowledging and examining our emotions is the only way to releasing that which does not serve us. So, we must not ignore our emotions whatever we do.

But our emotions do represent what is in the way. And our emotions have a cause within us. So that makes it simple. We must get at the cause. That's the only place we can effect a change. What causes these emotional states that block the connection to real cause?

Well, that's why I did that hard research with mama bear. We now know that fear - except when you are being chased by a bear - makes us do everything backwards. We got carried away with our emotions and let them take over our lives because we got carried away with fear to the point of letting it become the dominating factor in our lives. We gave fear so much prominence in our lives that it became our motivation. Of course, that can't work. Love is the only real motivator in the universe. We're not accomplishing much the way we are. We're not even doing a good job of looking after ourselves, let alone getting on with our job description.

Fear, not to mention hate, has sort of taken over our lives. And hate is just another form of fear of course. All negative emotions are derivative of fear so let's not waste time categorizing them. It's all fear.

So where did fear come from? From our sense of separation from source.

In the seeming absence of Love, something is not going to feel good. And that bad feeling boils down to fear no matter how you slice it. Any feeling that is not of Love is negative and takes something away from what we are. There is only Love. Therefore, fear can only be defined as an absence of Love. All negative emotions come from fear. So, our false prophet within is fear. Plain and simple. Again, that was the easy part, identifying the false prophet. The harder part is doing something about it.

Fear dictates most of our actions. It was fear that stopped me in my first try at total acceptance with my co-worker way back somewhere. I feared that I wouldn't get my work done. And yet, when I finally just gave up and said the hell with it - when I finally just got out of the way - Love was able to do its work and my work went much, much better. That's just one example. But if we want to take a long hard look at most of our everyday activities and really be honest about it, we will see that fear directs our actions at almost every turn. We can do better than that. A lot better.

All we have to do is turn ourselves inside out, which means dealing with fear head on. All we must do is find a way to stop using fear as a motivator. Self-examination and acknowledging comes to mind for starters. And yes, that's why that was covered so thoroughly earlier. So that's all good but it's time to get even more thorough and rid ourselves of this problem once and for all.

Everything works in harmony in our natural state. There are any number of things that work together that our bodies and minds may function harmoniously. An obvious physical example is how the body heals itself but there are many others. Dreams, as another example, are natural psychotherapy. That's how our minds are designed to self-heal. Everything about us is designed to function in literally

Divine harmony. Beings of Love quite naturally have a built-in corrective system to function perfectly.

And normally we never think about these things. There is no need. We just go about the business of living and take all these wonderful things for granted, if we think about them at all. We usually never come close to appreciating our own greatness. But when something goes wrong, we often do a little investigating to see if we can figure it out and do something about it. And that ability in itself is quite remarkable.

And something has gone wrong. Now I could just point out that we have left Love out of the mix, and that that's our whole problem. And I wouldn't be the first one to say that. We have songs, poetry, and endless reminders that Love is the all of everything. There was a very popular song by the Beatles, 'All you need is love.' If I remember right, there wasn't much more to the song. That was the main line in the song, and they mostly just kept repeating it. Good point. That is the simple truth. But we need details and specifics to affect a remedy. We have gotten just far enough away from Love that a simple reminder of its all-serving purpose doesn't seem to be quite good enough anymore. Or I could just say that we need to be at peace. Peace of course is the key to inviting Love's return. To be at peace is the open door to Love. Everybody knows that too. But that's also too general.

So it comes down to the simple fact that we are in a place where we have to break the process down and examine some of the details of how we function to see what went wrong. How did we get into a situation where we habitually leave the most important ingredient out of the recipe? We can see how we might have missed a few details here and there, but how on earth did we get to the point where we expect to make a cake with arsenic instead of sugar? Something is fundamentally wrong. So, we have no choice.

We have to look at the basics of how we function. It can be a little tedious but what else is there to do?

Quite a number of people got together and mapped the entire human genome. How's that for tedious? If we can do that, I'm sure we can spend a few minutes on what I am advocating here. That genome thing was an absolutely astounding accomplishment, but it still didn't tell us how Love keeps us functional. And I don't know that either of course. Divine Love is a big mystery to me. All I know is that it works. But I do know a little about some of the simple mechanics of the mind.

There is one in particular designed for us to have continuity of identity. And like everything else, it can't work without Love. And of course too, like everything else, without Love it continues to work but it can't do what it was designed to do without the main ingredient. It's an automatic process that will work as directed. So, if it's directed by fear it will work within the terms of fear. It will work very well to keep us stuck in fear as long as it is directed by fear. Let's take a look at that mechanism and its process and see if that helps.

This simple mechanism within our minds does its work by checking all new information against what is already established. This mechanism, like all the other automatic processes of our minds, works literally at the speed of light. So, we usually don't notice it. The speed of light is 186,000 miles per second, so for all practical purposes in our physical world, that's instantaneous. And another reason we don't notice this mechanism is that we aren't supposed to. It's just one of those things built into us that we need so that we can focus our attention on the business of living without a lot of tiresome details. Like a lot of repetitive tasks we put on computers nowadays to make life easier. But as I just mentioned, something has gone awry, so that compels me to go through this boring routine of checking it out and see if we can fix it and get back on track - get back to living life the way it was planned and the way the system was set up. We're on our own with this. God set it up perfectly, and if we want to mess with it with faulty commands, that's our problem.

What has gone wrong with that system that checks all incoming information for compatibility with that which is already established? No, that's not quite right. Nothing has gone wrong with the system. It continues to do its work with 100% efficiency and works as directed. It's the direction that's causing the problem. The system can't make the adjustment to work without Love. It wasn't designed that way. It wasn't designed to be directed by fear. Nothing was. So of course, that beautiful little mechanism, to repeat myself, works as directed. That mechanism that is designed to keep out all that is not compatible with established data is effectively your guardian at the gate. It guards against all incoming incompatible data so that you can stay sane. And it's still on the job. That's not the problem. But now it is the guardian of all the *erroneous* data it has learned to accept and therefore will not let in truth anymore.

We know how that happened. The mind did not acquiesce to doing things backwards without enormous rebellion of course. But it, the mind, had the terrible disadvantage of being in a little body when it was forced to buy the great lie. All the big people around this beautiful mind in a little body bombarded it with all that incompatible data until it finely gave up never to see truth again in this lifetime. That was the terrible two's I explained in the beginning and which I have expanded on since. So once that process of conforming to what is a fundamental error, is complete - once a child accepts enough erroneous data to where it reaches critical mass - that data takes the place of the original and perfect data that the child started out with. At that point the reversing process is complete. From there on, that famous mechanism I am referring to, checks all incoming information against that core of the new established data that has taken place of the original. Henceforth the guardian at the gate refuses entry to anything other than the fiction of the world. Worse, having paid such a high price for conformity, there is no way we will allow this reversal again. We have very effectively established such a strong emotional attachment to our false identity that we don't even want to think about looking at anything else.

That's the part I missed of course, as I have explained earlier. But thank God and psychiatry for schizophrenia or I would be in the same boat as everyone else. So, this is me still at the age of two, and only now rebelling and insisting on the truth and more. I am also insisting that this process of conformity can be undone. It can be undone by self-examination, the pursuit of peace, thoughtfulness and understanding and probably a few other things. We all have the ability to self-heal in every way, within ourselves. But we must activate the process. And that activation can only be done by deliberate conscious activity. The subconscious way we have been taught to live our lives will not and cannot work for the healing of our minds and bodies and our spirit.

For normal people this could be a challenge. But help is on the way. We need to tie this guardian at the gate thing in with something else to get on with healing; with another of our built-in abilities. We have another astounding ability. We have the profound ability to reflect and to self-examine. We can play back our own thought processes to ourselves. As mentioned, our thoughts go by very quickly, but we can actually stop and slow the process down and back up and examine what just went through our heads. This is not something you have to learn. We all do it all the time. And what that means is that we can examine and watch how that guardian at the gate works. We can break the process down one frame at a time and see just what's happening so that we can understand what has gone wrong. Then we can do something about it, to fix it. It is a most useful ability and the great saving grace that affords us the luxury of change.

I have noticed that if I have something wrong with the engine in my car, the mechanic asks me to start it so he can listen or otherwise observe. Let's do a little practice run with the mind and see if we can see why it's not running right. Assuming you don't like that knock or that ticking sound of course. Let's pour in some new information and see what happens.

Since we have clearly been given information that we are perfect beings, why not try something that fits that category. Like, 'I never make mistakes.' (If this is the truth for you, you don't need to be reading this). Now stop right there and play it back including the thought or thoughts that came up as the result of that statement. I can almost guarantee that you had thoughts that contradicted that statement. Well of course, you say, who wouldn't with a statement like that? And that's fine. This is just an experiment to examine this mechanism up close so that we can see if it works. So, the system works fine. It did indeed check the new against the old as it was supposed to. It rejected the information for lack of compatibility just like it was supposed to.

That was a look and a breakdown of two of the functions within us so that we can understand what went wrong. And that's the good news and the bad news. The bad news is that we have done a complete reversal as far as allowing data into the system that is life enhancing. The good news is that we have the ability to examine the process which means we can do something about it. But we still have one more key characteristic which is basic to our makeup to deal with. There is an important issue that must be dealt with before we can make any real change.

We are quite naturally emotionally attached to that data within us because it represents our present identity. So, we're back to emotions again. But if we recognize that most of our emotions have become our false prophet, we're on the way to solving the problem. Solving problems always starts with acknowledging what's wrong. So, if we start to look at our emotions with a critical eye, we can start to see ourselves very differently.

It can be very helpful when trying to understand a difficult problem to take it to an extreme - to highlight it so that we can have a better look at it and to try it on in an exaggerated form. We just happen to have such a state. I have had firsthand experience with an exaggerated form of emotionalism: The emotional state induced with alcohol. But I am not suggesting that you rush out and get drunk to verify this. I already did that for you and trust me on this; it's true. Alcohol is quite capable of taking our emotions to an exaggerated state.

I have put back a few beers in my time and I remember the state it put me in. Actually, I have memories of more than one occasion in this state. One could even say that my research on this topic has been thorough. I can't speak from the full authority of an alcoholic, but I do know what it's like to be drunk. And the thing I remember the most about drunkenness is how my emotional state would change considerably. And as a consequence, I would think and do things that I definitely would not do without the aid of alcohol. My reasoning process seemed to undergo a change, sometimes diminishing to the point of near zero. Most of my actions and behaviour were dictated by my emotions. I also remember rather liking that state to the point of conveniently forgetting the price one pays on the following day. I did in fact deliberately seek out this state that I might have experiences I would not otherwise have. Alcohol and emotions keep you coming back for more. So there really is not all that much difference between one who is hooked on alcohol and one who is hooked on emotional highs. But there is one huge difference in the likelihood of anyone seeing through the limitation that these states can keep us in.

With alcohol, you can't really lie to yourself. You have to know that this isn't working - many people do, and many people make a change. But living through our emotions is considered normal so we usually do not regard that as a problem, let alone do anything about it.

Alcohol removes inhibition enough so that we tend to act, do, and say things that we might not otherwise indulge ourselves in. But why the inhibitions to start with? What is there within us that we hold back in normal everyday living? How is it that we even have things that we don't express 'normally'? Well, that takes us right back to our fictitious world and polite society and what is politically correct. In other words, there is a big part of our world that isn't fit for expression, and we all know that and so we restrain ourselves. Alcohol removes that restraint at least to some extent and one is more apt to express what one 'feels'. Now I would under no circumstances advocate drinking, but sometimes there is more honesty involved with those who drink than we might see in other areas of society. If you don't count the incoherence of course.

As mentioned, one of the things that alcohol does is liberate a fair bit of the reason that would otherwise provide a certain check and balance to one's thought processes and behaviour. How liberating not to be weighted down with reason even for a short time. So, alcohol often reveals that which we deny, even if it is done in a rather rough sort of way. And it does so through our emotions - those emotions that come from that which is inherent in this world of make believe we have created.

Maybe that's why so many people drink. Our world is enough to drive you to drink. It is an unconscious attempt to release that which is not serving us. Drinking at least allows us to express. And expression certainly can be a beginning toward releasing and is very therapeutic. But the problem with this homemade therapy is that there is no real releasing done and therefore it nicely misses the point. It in fact, solidifies the very patterns that we are trying to release. So lest there be any misunderstanding, drinking doesn't work. The best it can do is shorten your life and thereby reduce your misery. Drinking is only an understandable reaction to the frustrating limitations of how we have learned to live, but it doesn't solve anything. It only makes things worse. Drinking is just a blind attempt at getting to our real knowing - that real knowing that is forever prodding us, wanting recognition.

Using the example of the state induced by alcohol, I am pointing out that some states exaggerate our emotions. I am told that no experience is ever wasted, even if we might wonder about this one. But let's try.

This state of mind reveals the stark reality of the perils of living by our emotions and the addictive nature thereof. This exaggerated form of emotionalism certainly points out the fallacy of any positive expectations in terms of enlightenment. One may very well *feel* enlightened, and even strongly believe that wonderful new insights have been gained, but somehow on the morning after, all these brilliant ideas just evaporate.

But that doesn't mean that those who don't drink are off the hook. Defining oneself by what one does not do is still defining oneself in terms of the world. Spirit is a little more demanding than that. If we need a standard to measure ourselves by, it was pointed out clearly some time back. None of us are immune from the conditions of the world. In fact, those who rate themselves as better because of what they don't do are probably in a worse trap than those who do these things because the need for change is hidden. The need for change is obvious for someone who drinks or uses drugs or otherwise indulges in methods to cope with the unsatisfactory ways of our world.

But here is what we need to know about emotional highs: The problem with emotional highs is that they contain their opposite. I know, we live in a world of opposites. And that sort of works for everyday life and we will cover that more thoroughly in the next chapter, but: But our spirit does not have opposites. Therefore, and again to put it simply, we must temporarily set aside our normal way of being when we seek to connect to our spirit.

First, I want to get clear on this business of emotional highs containing their opposite because it is the critical point of understanding this pitfall. Feeling low was our starting point from which we were able to induce a state of feeling high or why would we bother. This means that the starting point still exists. But since spirit does not have opposites and certainly does not have a starting point of feeling low, and since also, the entire purpose we are addressing here is the process of reconnecting to spirit, we cannot come at spirit from this standpoint. That platform of feeling low did not evaporate just because we used it as a springboard. The low and high cancel each other out in terms of making a permanent connection to spirit. Sorry about that but times up; we can't lie to ourselves anymore.

That's the catch with emotional highs. We get a glimpse of the real thing, our natural state, and we think we have arrived. We settle for these emotional highs as the real thing because they *are* the real thing. Our natural state *is* feeling good all the time. But what we are trying to do here is to go all the way with this, to grow beyond and therefore eliminate that which keeps us from our natural state. To in fact come to a place where we do indeed feel good all the time instead of for just a brief moment when we are propelled into an emotional high. That emotional high is a glimpse of our natural state, but it cannot be maintained as long as its opposite exists.

So, our false prophet is exposed: The fictitious self that we created while separated from Source. It will maintain itself in perpetuity as long as we settle for those highs because they have their base within the fictitious self. And it comes to us in sheep's clothing and is indeed a ravenous wolf. It's very easy to get sucked in. This imposter is very difficult to discern because, for just a moment, it is the same as the real thing.

Emotional highs can be induced with just a little hoopla, especially if you have a charismatic speaker to help you along. And 'oh wow' does that feel good. And you can always go back for more and it doesn't give you a hangover. So, what does this mean? It means that we must come at this in a different way if we want to facilitate a permanent change in consciousness.

We must refrain from any exercise that produces these temporary highs in our attempts of reconnecting to spirit. The true spiritual aspirant will no more allow an emotional high to define his spiritual progress than he would indulge in drugs or alcohol. We covered refraining in chapters 8 and 9 with the grand finale about fasting in chapter 10. And that was good but much more obvious than this issue. Here, this business of living in terms of what the outer world would dictate is not at all easy to see. It is so well hidden because our false prophet disguises itself so well. But there is a way to see through the disguise: ***Ye shall know them by their fruits.***... It's so simple really. What are the results? The fruits of your efforts. Did that sudden emotional realization produce some tangible result in your outer world?

I for one want to do whatever I can to get beyond that state which compelled me to take action that almost caused my demise in my little frolic with Mama bear. This is not freedom. It's more like a built-in self-destruct program. Which takes us to the obvious question: If we can't connect to spirit through emotion, how do we connect?

Through *feeling.*

So how do we deploy the feeling we lost from our disconnection to spirit when we are disconnected from spirit? There's that nice little conundrum or catch 22 that we always have in this endeavour.

Through peace.

It all starts with peace, with deliberately taking steps to create peace within ourselves. Whatever it takes to be in a state of peace, it's worth any price because it is our Divine connector to the Divine. That's our natural state, so to get back to our natural state we must cultivate our natural state.

Blessed are the peacemakers,
for they shall be called the children of God.

Our natural state as children of God is no worries, which is peace - no concerns of any kind because everything is provided for. ***Give us this day our daily bread.*** We covered that. We have the keys to the kingdom. A feeling of peace connects us to the ultimate feeling which is Love. And from there all is forthcoming because Love is the compatible software with all that is. To be ***called the children of God*** means to be referred to as we truly are - to be in our natural state. We need to practice being in our natural state to return to our natural state. We can't simplify it more than that.

So, to get back to connecting to spirit with feeling, we do indeed pursue spirit with feeling. We do not under any circumstances pursue spirit with indifference or a neutral attitude. The more intense the feeling the better. Feeling is our grand connector to spirit. But as mentioned, the character and quality of the feeling we are looking for has to be regained in our disconnected state. The feeling we are looking for is very different then an emotional high generated with ra, ra, ra. That's great for a cheerleading group but useless for what we are trying to accomplish here. Actually, it's worse than useless, a lot worse. But we have already covered that.

For anything else in life of course our emotional highs are what make us human. We enjoy that ecstatic state when the home team wins or any other success or for all the great things in life. All forms of recreation and special occasions are a celebration of being human. And of course, we should enjoy all these good things to the fullest. Our emotions define that enjoyment.

But settling for temporary highs in our pursuit of spirit is the ultimate tragedy. That high is truly and literally nothing compared to the perpetual state of Peace, Love, and Joy that is our natural heritage.

Chapter Seventeen

MATTER

*Not every one that saith unto me, Lord, Lord,
shall enter into the kingdom of heaven;
but he that doeth the will of my Father
which is in heaven.
Many will say to me in that day,
Lord, Lord have we not prophesied in thy name?
and in thy name have cast out devils?
and in thy name done many wonderful works?
And then will I profess unto them,
I never knew you:
depart from me, ye that work iniquity*

I once watched a really strange TV show. It was a story about a group of people who adhered to a religion based on the biblical quote on *faith, hope, and charity'*. Not a bad idea. That covers just about everything, and I can see how you could form a religion on that. But unfortunately, there was a misprint in their bible and the 'e' was missing from the word hope. So, these people hopped everywhere they went in obedience to the decree in their bible. The show was a little bizarre and I didn't watch the whole thing. I just clicked back to it occasionally during commercials in another show. But if there was a point to that show, I would guess it had something to do with thinking and possibly making use of the ability to reason. It seems to me that if just one person in the group had engaged his mind, it could have saved them a lot of trouble. But as I said, it was a very strange show. And it was very repetitive.

Strange and repetitive yes, but it is symbolic of how far from our own nature we have strayed - how far off we are in what we believe is required of us by God. God requires nothing from us or how would He have allowed us to proceed with this barbaric we interact? We have done, and are doing, some rather strange things in this state we are in - this state of separation in which we imagine ourselves as the matter that we came to dwell within.

This is why we have this grand finale of warnings about the hazards involved in this process of change. The straight and narrow got us on topic, pointing out the simple truth that the ways of the world are by far the strongest influence and that more of us than you might expect, could miss the turnoff. And that led us to the big one: That our false prophet, represented through our emotions, are the last bastion of survival for our false self; as wonderful as our emotions are, they can be extremely misleading. This is where the fictitious self takes a do or die stand. We do indeed have the ability to take in all this information only to enhance that fictitious self; which leads to this conclusive warning:

> ***Not every one that saith unto me, Lord, Lord, shall enter into the kingdom of heaven; but he that doeth the will of my Father which is in heaven***

Everything we have covered has suggested a flip in thinking. From loving our enemies to the big trap of judgment, just to mention a couple of the larger issues. And we've had quite a few clues about what the finished product is supposed to look like; our real identity has been spelled out for us. We've covered everything and we have all the information we need. We even reconciled the seeming contradiction of Thy will and my will. So now we have come full circle and are back to that first big therefore we ran across in chapter two:

As much as it is important, even critical, to have a clear understanding of all this, and therefore what we are all about, there is that crucial *doing* step involved: It is only by *doing* that there is value in what we have covered - to actually *do* these things until we *feel* it as real within us. It is only by putting these things into practice that they become recorded, imprinted, and ingrained in the subconscious. Only then are we able to express what we really want to express, spontaneously. We become capable of expressing our true selves again in every moment.

The ways we have adopted and how we have defined ourselves have become very heavily embedded. That's why we needed somebody to come along and give us a wake-up call. And it's just now starting to sink in after 2000 years.

And I thought I was slow!

As I said in the beginning, the ratio of time spent learning is way off. We spend far too much time getting the hang of this business of living life before we can get on with it which leaves us very little time at the end to enjoy life.

***

When I was about 7 years old, I got a bright idea. It was wintertime and my siblings and I had a few homemade sleighs that we played with. It was fun to ride a sleigh and slide down a hill. But that always required effort on somebody's part. The slide down the hill required walking up and riding on a sleigh in other areas required that somebody pull the sleigh. And that worked not bad. We took turns pulling. Mostly it was the bigger kids pulling the sleigh for the smaller kids. I was in the middle so I had a little of both.

I wondered if there could be a way to get around this business of pulling the sleigh, although that's certainly not the terms I would have used in my imaginings those days. Of course, my parents had solved that problem with horses. That seemed to work well. The horses pulled the big sleigh in the winter and the wagon in the summer. We even had a 'one-horse open sleigh' for social events. But all those things were adult things and I needed something that would work for me, for a child's sleigh. So, the bright idea came into my head to tie two sleighs together, sit on one, and push the other. And I did in fact follow through with my brainwave. I went to the trouble of tying two sleighs together and attempted to proceed as planned. I was very disappointed. But I got it. I understood why that couldn't work, even if I could not have put it into words like I might be able to now.

My little experiment was a source of great merriment for my older brother when he found out about it, but that's fine. He's the genius.

***

Science tells us that for every force there is an opposite and equal force. I got a little glimpse of that when I was 7 years old. Well yes, I understand now. How else could the structure of our physical universe exist? Everything we see has two forces to keep it in place. It works like a swinging door that opens both ways. The door is held in place by two springs. If one of the springs is stronger than the other, then the door will not be held exactly in place. It will be ajar to some extent. But the force that holds the physical universe together is much more reliable than a spring. The force that holds our physical world together is Divine and works perfectly all the time.

So that force, of course, is extremely powerful. It can't be haphazard or variable. It works: Guaranteed. And it's the same force that keeps our bodies together. So, because we live in our bodies, we feel that force - can't be avoided. It comes with the territory. That force is an influence. An all-pervading influence that can affect everything we think and do.

There are two opposing forces in our world. Everything has its opposite or the physical world couldn't exist. We have up and down, hot or cold, good or bad, strong or weak, night or day, and we even have life and death. Anybody could make a long list. Everything you can think about in the physical has its opposite. Two equal and opposing forces keep everything firmly in place. The two opposing forces I unknowingly engaged with my two sleighs kept me firmly in place as it was meant to, despite my different expectations.

So let's take that into the realm of thinking. Most of the examples I used above hold true for thinking. You can be happy or sad, kind or mean, truthful or deceitful, loving or hateful, good or bad, and let's not forget success and failure. Again, anybody could make a long list. This business of everything having an opposite seems to hold even within our minds and it pretty well describes the world we live in. We had a good look at that in the last chapter with how our emotions can keep us in one place. It would seem that in our world of this and that, we can't have one without the other. The influence of this and that suggests that we act and do things against the possibility of not being able to.

That's the nature of our physical world and it can keep us firmly in one place just like my sleigh experiment. Yes, that's the nature of physicality, but that's not *our* nature. This and that holds our world together and it even holds our bodies together, and it is how our brains function, but it is not what holds us together. There is an additional factor to consider, that, if you'll pardon the expression, makes all the difference in the world; when we consider our real nature, we need to consider this and that, *and* this other thing. We are not this and that. We *are* the other thing. We have an additional point of reference. And I'm sure everybody knows what that is by now. Have we not covered it at every opportunity? Love was always meant to be the dominating influence because it is our nature and it is the power with which we have been delegated to manage the 'this and that' of this world. Love is the power that commands every this and that, there is.

So if we concentrate exclusively on our physical nature, we must live in a world of limitation that keeps us more or less in one place. But everything we have been learning here is about our real nature and how it is not limited. And everything we have been learning has also been about how to get back to taking command of our lives and everything else in this physical realm, by getting back to that real nature. Our real nature is that which *encompasses* all of the laws of the physical world.

Therefore, we can take command of the 'this and that' of this world. Not that big of a deal, but it is what our entire topic is about. It is learning to take back our power by getting back to the truth about ourselves. It is about remembering our real nature so that we can work with and direct the 'this and that' of physicality, to our liking - transcending 'this and that'. We just forgot that all important detail about ourselves and so we let the strong influence of our physical nature control us instead of us taking control of it.

If we don't take command of our minds, our thoughts can keep us in one place too, just like my two sleighs did. Whenever we have a new thought, the structure of our brains immediately presents the opposite as a possibility. It has to. That's the nature of our physical brains. And that's very handy and useful. We can't do without it. It's the checks and balances, the constant feedback without which we would be *completely* dysfunctional. That's the only way we can live in our physical world, but as mentioned, our thoughts can keep us in one place with the greatest of ease unless we do something about it.

If we listen to the activity of our minds, we would never ever advance a new idea because of that opposite effect. The program we already have in place will simply tell us that it can't be done. But apparently, our thoughts are not keeping all of us in one place or how would anything new ever come into the world. We do make advances in thinking all the time, especially lately. We are going ahead with new ideas at such an astounding rate that they can make your head spin. In modern terms, that's called thinking outside the box.

And that's exactly the kind of thinking we have to adopt in this endeavour. We must think outside of the big box: That big box that has boxed us in for eons. But again, because 'this and that' has become the norm, some of us are a little reluctant to let go of it. It's challenging to entertain entirely new possibilities because that box has become our comfort.

So thinking outside of the box for what we have here is thinking outside of our normal identities. And that means questioning everything we have ever believed. And it means being open to even the most outrageous new possibilities - like entertaining the strange notion that we are perfect beings. That declaration wasn't just some far-off thing impossible to reach. That was the simple truth that had to be included in a final update and is meant to be taken seriously.

Our thinking is capable of going beyond the box by the very reason that we have the ability to think. We are consciously aware which means that we are the thinking part of the universe. And as has been so carefully explained, creation is directed by thought. But without that knowledge of ourselves, the 'this and that' of our world must dominate our thinking. And that dominance is experienced as fear, which as we now know is an absence of Love. And of course, an absence of Love is the absence of the very essence of what we are. The absence of Love is the absence of our power.

Back to my failed experiment with my two sleighs. I can't quite leave that alone. With my apologies to my older brother, I still believe we can go beyond the limitations suggested by the results of my little test. No one has expected greatness from me since that little episode, but I haven't given up that there might still be a way to pull it off. Maybe I was onto something there and just didn't have the maturity to understand it. It's safe to say that I had not developed my reasoning faculties back then. So where did this bright idea come from? Why would such an unreasonable idea come into my mind when it's obvious that it was a rather futile, if not an infantile exercise? I don't believe nature is that wasteful and I don't believe ideas come from nowhere. Rather, I believe that the idea came to me because it was consistent with a greater truth. And it came to me because I wasn't burdened with reason. Back then, my mind wasn't developed to the stage that I was able to reason it through to the point that it would have saved me the trouble of the experiment. And my mind still isn't developed to the stage where it will accept reason without question and it's extremely unlikely that it will ever be. Now I realize that I am making a case for schizophrenia here - giving validity to my condition. But I'm coming out of the closet and I demand equal rights.

It's obvious to me that reason is highly overrated. As I have already pointed out, reason can cancel any new idea because everything has its opposite. So I'm back to that question: How do new ideas come into existence in this world? Too obvious by now, I would guess. By giving up reason. How else? Which as mentioned is called thinking outside of the box - entertaining entirely new possibilities, even radical departures from the norm. Most will not work and will in fact, probably be laughable, but who cares. If we have one new idea at the end of the day, one new thing that works and has never been done before, the world is better off. So what all this means is that we are capable of giving up reason and still be functional. In fact, when it comes to introducing new ideas, the only reason to use reason is to make sure it makes sense. What we call creative thinking does not come from reason. Reason is usually the big inhibiting factor to creative thinking.

So to get back to my little experiment, let's look at what I was really trying to do. It's simple. I was trying to get something for nothing. All that business of walking up a hill so I could slide down, or forever trying to get someone to pull the sleigh, didn't seem right to me somehow. And as I have already indicated, the reason it didn't seem right to me is that I was not yet bogged down with reason. And I was right. There is something for nothing. The natural way is that everything is free and I knew that, way back then. It's just that the way of the world did not present a framework within which my needs were readily forthcoming. I just didn't know how to go about getting what I wanted then. And I still don't. But it's not my fault if we made up a world with all these crazy limitations. The way the world is set up right now, it's very difficult to get something for nothing. But that doesn't mean that it can't be done. I insist that my idea was, and is, valid. I just haven't arrived at a place in creative thinking that has allowed it to happen yet, that's all. And it might be a while before I do. But there are people in the world who are exploring fascinating new concepts about energy. It is only just lately that we are finding 'free' energy in the world. We're getting there. The day is coming when we will understand the full implication of, **give us this day our daily bread**.

Still, the influence of our physical world can cause us to use reason beyond reason and to inhibit the flow of our real knowing. We can get so involved with what we think we know that we do not invite the new into our lives. The up and down, hot and cold, good and bad and the 'this and that' of our world can dominate our thinking to the point of not even understanding each other; so much so that we end up with a lot of seemingly irreconcilable differences. We even take our misunderstandings to the extreme of killing each other. Taking the influence of 'this and that' to that extreme is of course losing all semblance of the reality of our nature. So we do have to take that influence seriously. It's very powerful and can lead us to our destruction.

That we might take that influence and our subsequent sense of separation and our identification with our bodies to that extreme, was probably not imagined, even by God. The only possible good thing about getting that far off the mark is that it tells us how powerful the influence of our 'this and that' world can be. The influence of the force that holds all matter together has just been too much for us to handle. We have allowed this influence to be so much a part of us that it has overridden most of the influence of the Divine within us. With that strong influence, we have forgotten what matters.

When we say something doesn't matter, we mean it is of no importance and nothing to worry about. But we use the word matter in another sense too. Matter is what makes up all things of the earth and all physical objects. We refer to the matter that makes up anything in our world, right down to play dough. Yet we use this same word to indicate the relative importance of almost everything we think or do. And we say things like, 'what is the matter with you', which seems to indicate that we are too ensconced in matter. So the real question then is: Does matter really matter all that much? It seems to. But surely it doesn't matter to the degree we have taken it to. We need to get things in perspective to understand what really matters. And we have that ability. We can increase our understanding of ourselves and get it all in proper balance.

And the most interesting thing about that process is that as we gain a larger perspective, the things that once were important become less important or even insignificant; the larger the perspective the less anything matters. So how high can we go when it comes to getting a larger perspective? Is there a perspective large enough with which to view matter where matter might not matter at all?

Well yes, of course there is. And that just happens to be a key to understanding matter a lot better. That understanding starts with seeing ourselves in a very different light. When we begin to grasp the concept that we are not matter at all - when we begin to know the real truth about ourselves, that our real essence is spirit - then the matter that our bodies are made of matters a little less. It's still important; our bodies are the temples for our spirits, so they are very important. But our bodies are not something we can't do without. We just can't function in this world without them, that's all.

So to get started with real understanding we need to consciously address this question like my grandson did. What am I? The all-important question. He couldn't possibly know the full significance of his question at that time and certainly not of the answer, but at least he asked it. There is much, much more to my answer when he is ready to ask it and there is much, much more to us whenever we are ready to hear it.

But in the meantime, just so we get a bit of an idea of what we truly are, we can look at what we are not. We are not just our bodies. Our bodies are made up of matter but as we all know by now, that's not all there is to us. Matter is creation and we are part of that. More than a part, we are the knowing part of creation. We represent Creator within creation.

So matter *is* important. More than important, matter is sacred because it is creation. And our bodies are very important as physical creations. But to get so caught up with matter to the point that nothing else matters, is definitely going too far. I don't think matter matters at all when we are dead. I'm sure that when we pass on, we view this whole matter thing very differently.

But that's not to say or in any way infer that we should not take our experience here seriously. The physical universe is indeed absolutely sacred, the beauty of which is beyond description in human terms. But to enjoy this awesome beauty, we need to back away just a little - as you do with an oil painting. An oil painting looks kind of rough when you look at it up close, but when you stand back a bit, the real beauty comes out. So we need to stand back a bit from this business of being physical otherwise we can't really appreciate it. Getting too involved with creation takes the fun out of it.

If we get so caught up with creation that we actually identify our entire selves with it, we can't possibly enjoy it. You enjoy the painting because you see the beauty of it. The beauty is there to behold. Matter is meant to be the material with which we create and to behold, not that with which we identify ourselves. There is a larger perspective in which we see the beauty of ourselves *reflected* as matter, but that does not mean seeing ourselves *only* as matter. Otherwise, matter matters way too much.

The essence and the beauty and the completeness of what we are can never be replaced; only reflected. We have reflected ourselves in matter that we might enjoy creating and interacting within created matter. But real enjoyment cannot take place if we forget who we are. That's like going to a movie and getting so caught up in the drama that you identify with the characters. And that's fun and a good thing to do and we do that deliberately. But we also know that we can shut our eyes and remember who we are at any moment. And that was the whole idea of this drama here on earth. We just got so caught up in it that we forgot that we can stop and remember who we are at any moment. We forgot the ultimate larger perspective which would make the whole thing the greatest and ultimate joy.

We came here as co-creators to express ourselves as matter and to create *within* matter, so that we could be hands-on with an actual experience of what matter feels like. That was the great Divine idea that we agreed on. But we got so enamoured with matter that we forgot our Divine essence and therefore forgot the original plan. We came here to represent God complete with all the qualities of God. That's why God can't interfere when something goes wrong. Even terribly wrong - like the savagery of war for example. God can't interfere because we *are* God in action within creation.

The original plan was a little like a man going to the moon rather than just sending a satellite to orbit and take pictures. To be on-site - to be away from home, to explore first hand, and send new information back - is an astounding accomplishment. But that's where what we are doing is a little more than visiting the moon. We came here with much more than exploration in mind; we came here to create.

But this experience has been so distracting and we got so caught up in the process that we ended up mistaking the process for what we are; the means has become the end. And the final irony of it all is that only the most powerful of souls are capable of something like that. Only entities with complete autonomy and full creative abilities, could accomplish what we have done. If we had anything less than 100% jurisdiction over ourselves and this project, there would have been an intervention.

But forgetting what we are did not take away our Divine abilities. Only with that amazing 'accomplishment' of identifying ourselves with matter have we been able to see ourselves as separate from God. And that seeming separation has left us with the capability of using our Divine abilities for purposes other than Divine purposes; for any and all things unlike our own real nature. ***Verily I say unto thee, ye are Gods, and all of you sons of the most high!***

So here's the problem. Because we have identified ourselves with matter a little too exclusively, any attempt by an outside influence, or any information we receive contrary to our self-made identity only drives us deeper into that identification. And it does so because of the fragility of that identification. It takes constant support on our part to keep our fiction alive and that support quite naturally kicks in stronger whenever it is threatened - whenever we have evidence to the contrary. We are being bombarded with the truth these days. It's all around us. But you have to look for it. It won't come out and grab you for the very reason I just mentioned. We must do that on our own. We must ask or it cannot be given to us.

Except with what I am doing. This is where I have taken a different stand. I'm just crazy enough to deal with this problem head-on. I promised to be explicit because we can't afford to beat around the bush. The situation in the world is getting critical. Time's up. We are at a point where we are either going to get this or not. We need to look at everything we have available to us so that we can figure it all out. So I for one, am no longer holding anything back. Even our dysfunctional states have something to say about our condition in general. There was always a failsafe built into the system so that if we did happen to take our foray into matter to the extreme of forgetting, a time would come when it must end. How could it be that we would be left in this state in perpetuity? And of course, that time is now or how would I be able to tell you about it.

We are awakening from that mistaken identity we fell into. That's why there is so much commotion going on in the world. But what a grand celebration it will be when the transition is over and we remember. When we remember and see what we have done, we will see all that enormous and unbelievable hardship we endured in a vastly different way and we will put it all to good use. We might even say it was worth it. We could not have had this unique experience if we had not forgotten about ourselves.

But it *is* time to remember that we have the Divine ability to create and that all the necessary material has already been supplied. There *is* something for nothing. Everything is for nothing. We are just starting to find that out now and it is being demonstrated. Like solar and wind power for example. This means there is a way I can power my little sleigh and get a free ride. Everything is provided that we can just enjoy. That's what God would have us do - express the joy of living at all times. That's what we are all about as free spirits. Matter is truly beautiful, the ultimate beauty because it is the creation of the ultimate Creator.

My little experiment with my sleighs and the people that hopped everywhere on that TV show are about on par. There was a major misunderstanding and a lack of information in both cases. I think I should be let off the hook for my error because it was based in truth. But not so for our fictitious group in the television show. And apparently, none of us are off the hook if we misunderstand the simple requirement of getting reconnected to the source of our being.

All we have to do is exercise our God-given ability to think. We have been given the ability to ponder and question and try something different and even to think about what we are thinking about. And we have the ability to: **'Be still and know that I am God'**. We have the ability to do all these things until we awaken to our truth. And we have the ability to quietly and naturally put this truth into practice.

The great beauty of it all is that as complete autonomous beings, we each can expand creation in our own unique way. And that pleases God because God gets to have a new experience that He couldn't have any other way. As I said before, God loves surprises. And what we did is one big surprise even if it has been a royal pain at times.

How we have defined ourselves is not valid. We can't get to where we are going and take our fictitious selves with us. We are here to be. But we can't even get on topic, let alone address that question if we let the 'this and that' of our world dominate us.

We were meant to enjoy matter with abandon, but not to abandon ourselves to matter.

Chapter One

THE LIGHT OF THE WORLD

Blessed are the poor in spirit: for theirs is the kingdom of heaven.
Blessed are they that mourn: for they shall be comforted.
Blessed are the meek: for they shall inherit the earth.
Blessed are they who do hunger and thirst after righteousness:
for they shall be filled.
Blessed are the merciful: for they shall obtain mercy.
Blessed are the pure in heart: for they shall see God.
Blessed are the peacemakers:
for they shall be called the children of God.
Blessed are they who are persecuted for righteousness' sake:
for theirs is the kingdom of heaven.
Blessed are ye, when men shall revile you, and persecute you,
and shall say all manner of evil against you falsely,
for my sake.
Rejoice, and be exceeding glad:
for great is your reward in heaven:
for so persecuted they the prophets which were before you.

Ye are the salt of the earth:
but if the salt have lost his savour,
wherewith shall it be salted

It is thenceforth good for nothing,
but to be cast out, and to be trodden under foot of men.
Ye are the light of the world.
A city that is set on a hill cannot be hid.
Neither do men light a candle, and put it under a bushel,
but on a candlestick;
and it giveth light unto all that are in the house.
Let your light so shine before men,
that they may see your good works
and glorify your Father
which is in heaven.

    Walking up mountains is one of the many childhood habits that I have kept. There was one particular mountain that I walked almost daily for several winters. I had a circular route near the top that kept me from backtracking for at least part of the hike. I frequently saw tracks in the snow other than my own, although they were rarely human tracks. What I usually saw were the tracks of wild animals. After some time, one set of tracks caught my attention more than the rest. They seemed to be coyote tracks, which was no big deal. But the reason they caught my attention was that these tracks took a route similar to my route that made the circle. I never did see that coyote but I felt a certain affinity with it after a time because - if you will pardon the expression – we had common ground. I watched for the tracks and took note after a fresh snowfall to see how recent his travels might have been. This went on for a couple of months. I felt like I had a sort of friend that I had never seen, although it wouldn't have surprised me if he saw me. I'm sure this creature was more alert to his surroundings than I was, which wouldn't have been hard to do because I spent most of my time lost in thought.

My routine of walking always took place a short time after breakfast and breakfast always included at least two cups of coffee. I never gave a thought to bodily needs on the way up the mountain, but usually, after about 100 yards on the way down, the different impact of walking downhill seemed to affect my bladder and I would become aware of the need to relieve myself.

And, as mentioned, I have retained a lot more than the habit of walking up mountains from childhood. One of the simplicities with which a child might amuse himself, and that I kept over, was taking advantage of the requirement of emptying my bladder to make inscriptions in the snow. There is nothing like making marks in the snow for one easily amused. Normally I would have written my name or something like that, but for some strange reason, I took a different stance this time. Since it happened that my body demanded attention about the same place every day, it became a sort of ritual for me to make my mark in precisely the same spot every day. I took pride in a certain accuracy. A new snowfall was always a special occasion that necessitated the renewal of that same opening through the snow even if the previous marking was evident only by a vague indentation. Now anybody who knows anything about nature is aware that something has to give here. I was about to learn a very elementary lesson most dramatically.

As I approached my special spot and prepared to engage in my ritual, a very unusual sight glared out at me. My spot had been completely excavated and totally destroyed. Chunks of yellow snow scattered all over the place, along with a splattering of coyote tracks. Although that surprised me, there was something that caught my attention even stronger. This is where the dramatic part comes in. An emotional charge surrounded the area. It was so powerful that it overwhelmed my senses. Believe me, you didn't have to be psychic to get the message.

That wild animal was so offended by what I had done, that he was completely outraged. He must have been aware of my little stunt for some time and this awareness finally reached critical mass. I don't know, maybe wild animals have a certain respect for humans and that's why it took so long before he took the measure that he did, but whatever it was, his reaction was extremely powerful.

No animal would ever do what I had done. No wild animal would ever pee in the same place for starters. They of course use that for territorial markings among other things. But much more importantly, no wild animal would ever desecrate mother earth in this way. The earth quite naturally absorbs and recycles waste. BUT NOT ALL IN ONE PLACE!! That was such an outrageous violation to the earth as to be beyond belief. My coyote friend, if I still had a friend (He must have lost interest in any friendship long before his outburst. Who would befriend anyone who could be so departed from reality?), O.K., my ex-friend then, represented the outrage of mother earth herself and did a very good job of being her spokesperson. Believe me, I got the message, and never have I done anything like that since. I can feel the effects of that emotional charge to this day.

That coyote taught me something very valuable. Not bad for a creature without the ability to think, without a conscious mind with which to question the meaning of life. That's good communication skills for a life form that has no concept of language, let alone the ability to understand what a concept is. I would probably be considerably better off if I employed such basic wisdom in my everyday life.

Wild animals are a part of nature, living in harmony with the earth and with other creatures. Where any disharmony builds up, like overpopulation, for example, nature takes care of it. There are natural cycles of change essential to the harmony of the earth. No big mystery there. Everybody knows about that and we just accept it and call it natural. Wild animals work in ultimate harmony with nature because they don't have any other choice - in more ways than one. Choices that bring disharmony, like overpopulation, bring about an imbalance in food supply that nature must correct. So choices animals make are dictated by the environment and limited to their instinct. Anything more than that requires a conscious mind which they do not have.

And that's where we come in. We do have a conscious mind. That's what defines us as human and separates us from animals. We can make choices and then make further choices from those choices, and change our minds and start all over again. It's obvious that there is no limit to the choices we can make and what we can accomplish. And apparently, we can even make choices that are out of harmony with nature.

We can choose to do something repetitiously until it becomes habit. A habit is something we do automatically, subconsciously. And that's fine and good; it's part of what we are and how we function. We couldn't possibly get through the day without doing most things subconsciously. But now we are back into the domain of the animals. They do everything subconsciously for the simple reason that they don't have a conscious mind. The difference for an animal is that their lives are more or less set and somewhat predictable, at least from our point of view. They live by instinct. So when we create a habit we are effectively creating our own instinct. Now that's power! Especially when you consider that we have the ability to reverse that process if we don't like the results. We can get a whole new habit going until we do it automatically/instinctively. In other words, we can do pretty much whatever we want and we can also become so busy that we can forget that we have the option of making these major changes. We can form the habit of not considering some of the things we do habitually. And we can even let ourselves believe that we can get away with working out of harmony with nature.

I'm not trying to break new ground or give out new information just yet. All this is common knowledge. I'm just getting on topic so far. I am leading up to something and I want to be sure we agree on - some basics in case you want to leave before I take up too much of your time.

I would like to point out that some of our habits could use a second look. I'm sure that's no surprise either. But there is something bigger going on here. Most of the habits we have adopted as a mindset, or beliefs if you like, have been handed down to us from generation to generation. And that would be fine, but some of them aren't working so well. That business of conforming to our culture and general belief system is okay, but we don't have to do that. There is a strong influence to do so, but it is not compulsory. If we don't question these things, we are effectively giving up that which defines us. As we learn to conform, we sort of forget that we have all these choices; we effectively forget who we are. We function somewhat like the animals but without the innocence that allows nature to take care of us. Animals mostly make good choices because of the limitations of their instinct. They don't know how not to.

Nature takes care of us too, and in the same way, by the choices we make. But if we happen to have made some less than optimum choices somewhere in history and then made further less than optimum choices based on those former choices because that seemed like the only options available, we could be on a downward spiral. In other words, we are capable of functioning at a lower level than the animals even though we are vastly superior. And we have. Unless of course, I'm the only one who did something so dumb that the earth and one of her creatures had to create a dramatic scene to get my attention. But I'm keeping myself busy writing down some of my thoughts under the assumption that a few other people have made some blunders along the way as well. Even if those blunders may not have been quite that far off.

I have a conscious mind which renders me unlimited. My abilities cannot be compared to that of an animal. Yet I forfeited that sacred divine right to the point that I had to have a powerful wake-up call from a simple creature that does not have the ability to think. Surely I can do better than that. That's definitely not functioning at the optimum level. So I think we could do with some changes. But since each of us has complete autonomy, our general situation can only be changed by each person making a change. We do have complete freedom, but what each of us does, affects everybody else. We're all in this together.

The animals have a natural state and so do we. Because of our unlimited ability and freedom of choice, it is our nature to create a world of absolute peace, harmony, abundance, and any other good thing we can imagine. We can choose to form habits - do things instinctively - that are vastly different than what we are currently experiencing. It is natural for us to create heaven on earth. We just forgot our nature that's all. But we happen to have a reminder here, of how to get back to that real nature.

That explanation starts with an overview. But there is one more thing I need to point out before we get into that, just to make sure we agree on our agenda. There are a couple of quotes that pretty well cover where I'm coming from: *'As a man thinketh in his heart, so shall he be.'* And: *'Ye are Gods, and all of you sons of the most high, and the scriptures cannot be broken.'* The first quote indicates that what and how we think is what takes place in our lives. The last quote tells us what we are, and the fact that this is not changeable. Not much wiggle room there. No buts. But I will enlarge and clarify because that's what I'm doing here.

As a man thinketh is what these opening statements are all about. The implication is that we can do something about our thinking if we don't like what's coming down - a change in heart to cause a more favourable result. To that end and as a start, we can cultivate the habit of examining our thoughts. I read somewhere that a life unexamined is a life not worth living. Not only is a life unexamined not worth living, but it can be a little hazardous given the nature of the thoughts that some of us entertain. Therefore, self-examination is essential as a prerequisite to facilitating the release of anything unwanted before we start the process of accepting that which is more desirable.

But there is a tricky spot in the process of adopting a new mindset. Our consciousness is made up of thought patterns and beliefs that we entertain habitually and for which we have feeling. Feeling is the power. But it takes familiarity to establish feelings. A new ideal is like a new friend; feelings for someone new in your life usually comes only after you spend some time with and get to know that person, which takes us to the tricky part. Old friends sometimes don't get along with new friends but the old friends have the power because of the established feelings.

So in this process of change, it is essential to be protective of our new thought friends while we are establishing a relationship. And for sure we can expect rebellion from the old but that's part of the process. Even though the old have the advantage of being well established, our new friends have a quality that nobody can compete with: The new we are trying to introduce here are your Divine friends. Holding to that simple truth can get us past all challenges.

Which takes us to ***Ye are Gods***.

We are indeed. Yes, that's true and unchangeable, but apprentice Gods would actually describe us better in the stage we are in. That's one of the reasons we are referred to as children of God. As apprentice Gods, we have not yet learned how to exercise our full power. As children, we've just been playing at creating. We've been using playdough for the learning process. But the material that God uses to create is Love. So if we want to grow up and work with God, we have to learn to work with the real thing. It's not all that hard, but it can take a little practice.

We forgot the reality of what we are to get fully ensconced in this experience of being physical. We did a really good job but we got a little carried away. We got carried away to the point of neglecting and forgetting that critical part of us that is not physical. We forgot our real natures, which means we forgot Love among other things. Only through the seeming absence of Love could we possibly forget that we are Gods. And only through a seeming absence of Love could we possibly forget that it is through our thoughts that we make the great connection to the Divine, to creativity.

We've been creating more or less without an understanding of cause – Love - and that's why it's been so messy. And that's why this is such a big shift that has required a millennium or two to get on topic.

But that's what's changing in the world right now. This information age we are in is a reality check. It is time. And the information I have suggests that now is the time to get the full meaning of these old biblical quotes.

Okay, the opening statements: All of them have one big thing in common. Each one suggests very favourable results from a particular state of mind. These and the final openers about the salt of the earth and the light of the world give us a pretty good idea of where we are going with all this.

Blessed are the poor in spirit:
for theirs is the kingdom of heaven.

Our consciousness in biblical times was referred to as a kingdom because everybody understood the power of a king in those days. Our consciousness is our power centre. What we have established within ourselves as our beliefs and thought patterns, which become a part of us through feeling, defines our power and determines our experience. The terms are not important. What counts is that the power at our command cannot be overstated and that's why our consciousness is referred to as a kingdom.

And the very first recommendation on how to run the kingdom is to be ***poor in spirit***. To be poor in spirit is to have little in the way of spiritual knowledge or to be flexible with what we believe - a critical starting point. Since we are now looking for a complete understanding of ourselves, let's start over. Let's assume we know nothing; so much easier that way; so much easier to be open to something new. In other words, to be poor in spirit is to have an open mind. Any attempt at getting an understanding of how everything works can only start with an open mind. And an open mind is where a relationship with God starts. Therefore, our kingdom when it is open and focused on matters of the spirit is ***the kingdom of heaven***. The kingdom of heaven is a relationship with God.

This takes me back to those questions near the end of the prologue: Where do we start? Where do we begin with this business of getting a new approach to life that will lead us to a better definition of life? Well, this seems like as good a place as any to begin the beginning. How else might we start but with an open mind?

> ***Blessed are they that mourn,***
> ***for they shall be comforted.***

In case there was any doubt about the value of an open mind, this declaration should fix that problem. The definition of mourning as we use it here puts an open mind to the test.

The first part of the process of learning how life works includes noticing what doesn't work. As we look to higher truths, we will find these to be in opposition or contradictory to some of our old assumptions. We will find ourselves in a position of having to invalidate some old ideas or even cherished beliefs. In effect, part with dear old friends for whom we have strong feeling. That will cause mourning.

There are three stages to the mourning process: Denial, anger, and acceptance. All are necessary, but especially acceptance. It is only through acceptance that we can truly mourn because acceptance comes through acknowledgment. Acknowledgment starts when denial ends. Then anger takes over and the process ends with full acceptance. Only through the acceptance of loss is the mourning process complete. So there is a little more to acceptance than we might expect. There is a very important point here that is worth a little more attention. So I need to borrow a phrase used elsewhere to make that point.

I have been told that consideration for value in real estate rests with three conditions: Location, location, and location. I don't know much about real estate, but I do know that the value of learning comes only from three things in how we relate to anything undesirable that we are trying to release. To acknowledge, acknowledge, and acknowledge. Without acknowledgment, we have no chance at change. Without acknowledgment, the past can only stay with us indefinitely. Acknowledgment is the beginning of change. And we can expect to encounter that process with what we are doing here, and it is indeed a blessing.

We will be in the position of finding a lot of our old ways and beliefs to be invalid, to effectively realize we have been in denial. From the standpoint of our divinity, we are clearly in denial. There is no other way to handle living a lie. But as that denial becomes exposed, that open mind is put to the test. We will have the challenge of having to look at and release old beliefs that we have become attached to. There can only be mourning in such a process. To acknowledge and release that which once seemed so important because it was a part of us, will cause sorrow. Without sorrow, there can only be denial which means that

that which requires releasing is still in place. Mourning as we use the term here is complete acknowledgment.

Mourning may not be fun, but I don't know of a way of avoiding it without missing everything we are trying to accomplish here. This is a key to reconnecting. Without mourning, nothing new can be introduced. The blessing comes when acceptance and acknowledgment are complete. As the mourning process is completed, the new is integrated, which is the comfort.

Blessed are the meek:
for they shall inherit the earth.

Some of us have been overlooking our heritage for a long, long time. We have become preoccupied and have allowed our attention to be focused just about everywhere except toward Source - the source of our being. That preoccupation with outer things has become so extreme that it has caused us to forget how things work. We have been overlooking the cause in cause and effect. All that stress and strain we go through while we are busy wearing ourselves out trying to get what we want, doesn't work.

But then, that's what we are doing here. Getting back on track by finding out how things work. Remember the old adage: If all else fails, read the instructions. All else has failed, so there's nothing to do but read these instructions and see if we can assemble the pieces and reclaim our heritage.

To inherit the earth is to have jurisdiction. We have complete autonomy. The management of the conditions on earth has been delegated to us. And with that comes the power, resources, and freedom to manage as we will. Not to mention responsibility. To have command over all the conditions and circumstances of our lives here on earth is a given. We don't have to do anything to acquire it, except maybe quit trying so hard.

And not trying so hard can be quite a turnaround. We try too hard because things don't seem to come easy. And things don't come easy because we try too hard. But maybe by the time we are through with this little endeavour, we will see that there is an easier way; much easier.

A quiet, unassuming, humble, and even acquiescent stance in life is a radical change in focus. Yet, it is the change that addresses cause where cause really is; and therefore, opens the door to receiving. To be meek is to look with in - to look to Source to get connected to real power. There is no assertiveness or forcefulness involved at all; it's more like allowing. It takes character to be meek. It requires courage, strength, perseverance, patience, intelligence, and probably a few other things - the human spirit at its best. To be meek is to take back command of your life.

Our real power is within. Dominion is our true heritage. We have only to accept it by being focused on it. All things come from within, from Spirit, from God. When we acknowledge the source of our being, that power loves to manifest our desires. Even better, lovingly acknowledge if you want to pick up the pace. Better still, we can lovingly acknowledge our heritage with gratitude. That attitude acknowledges the source and makes the connection. We receive; we inherit that which is already given. Meekness is looking within for cause rather than trying to forcibly rearrange things in the outer world (but much more on this to come; this is just the overview).

Blessed are they who do hunger and thirst
after righteousness:
for they shall be filled.

Is there a point to all this? Is this just a should? Are we supposed to do all these things to be Godly people? And if so, is there some kind of reward or benefit? Or do we do this out of fear? Do we expect a reward after we die? Is this the requirement for getting into heaven? No, to all the above except the first one. None of the other things are motivators for one thing. But yes, there is a point and a reason to be motivated. Getting rid of pain, misery, and hardship are some of the reasons that come to mind. But aside from that, there are laws of the universe involved.

We work with and make use of the law of gravity in pretty well everything we do. Most people respect the law of gravity and we know that it is very dependable. Nobody has a gun to your head. You can ignore the law of gravity if you like but it won't ignore you. It's that simple. *That's* what this is for: To learn spiritual laws. These spiritual laws are just as demanding as the law of gravity and just as invisible and just as dependable. Can you imagine the mess if gravity took a day off?

We can learn about the laws of spirit just like we learned about the law of gravity as toddlers by falling off a chair, or we can make use of the greater abilities we have adopted since childhood and be a little easier on ourselves. We can become familiar with these laws and then learn by practice. We can try them out in the little things first until we gain confidence, and then pick up the pace and get these laws working for us to make our lives immeasurably better. More than better, we can go all the way with this and redefine life. That's the point.

So it helps to know that enough effort will get us there. If our desire is strong enough, we will get it right. What happens is, as we run these Truths through our minds and practice them, there is a build-up that increases until one day it reaches critical mass. The strength of the new has become strong enough to override and cancel out the old programming and suddenly you *are* the Truth. Then you wonder how you could have lived all that time without this connection to your real Self. Of course, this new state of being will require a little maintenance for a while to stabilize. And that's very important, essential actually, but it's nothing compared to the previous work.

So we have been given a word of encouragement here in case anyone finds this learning curve a little trying somewhere along the way. Those old ways that insist on recognition will atrophy with a persistent focus on what you know is right. A strong desire to get it right (righteousness), will prove to be a blessing. You will be filled with understanding, satisfaction, and well-being. You will get results. The system works.

Blessed are the merciful:
for they shall obtain mercy.

This one doesn't want a lot of explanation at this point, but it does contain a very powerful Truth. What we entertain in our minds towards others, is quite naturally, what comes back to us. This is about cause and effect and about forgiveness. Forgiveness is a really big issue and sometimes hard to understand not to mention implement. It is a cornerstone of these instructions and is fully covered later on.

Blessed are the pure in heart:
for they shall see God.

Starting with an open mind, fully acknowledging all that must be released, learning the true meaning of inner strength, developing a strong desire for the Truth, and finding forgiveness within ourselves is a process of releasing all of the negative from the subconscious. A process of purifying until there is nothing left to see but our Divinity.

Blessed are the peacemakers:
for they shall be called the children of God.

To make peace in your own mind is a big accomplishment. But whether it's a small job or a major cleanup, it is worth whatever it takes. It's cheap at twice the reward. Inner peace is the expressway to spirit. Spirit is constantly trying to communicate with us but the only reason it doesn't get through is because of a busy signal. Our minds are way, way too busy. It is of vital importance that we shut our minds off at least once in a while. We need to get out of our minds; stop thinking. Otherwise, nothing new can get through and we can only repeat.

Most of us have no terms of reference for real inner peace. I would go as far as to say that many of us have not known real peace since infancy. This world can be a little disturbing. So to get back to our natural state, we have to back off and spend time alone. The practice of the above states of mind contributes to peace and vice versa. If you can find peace, it is infinitely easier to assume those other states of mind. Peace is the rock, the state of all states to be desired and coveted. To still the mind, to experience silence within, is a sure way to connect. So to deliberately cultivate peace is truly to invite all blessings. Peace is our natural state. So the practice of peace can take us back to our natural state - to our real identity (again, much more on this later).

***Blessed are they which are persecuted
for righteousness sake,
for theirs is the kingdom of heaven.***

This ties in with peace. That wasn't hard to figure out. All these openers tie in with one another. Each one enhances the previous and contributes to the whole.

All of our endeavours - all the way to and especially including working toward peace - invites opposition. The mind rebels against new friends. Installing the new is going to stir things up a little. Programming new information into the subconscious mind is going to cause conflict with the old.

The subconscious mind is our faithful servant, automatically performing duties that we experience as habits - be they of a physical nature or in the way of established thought patterns. But the subconscious must have consistency. It cannot accept information that is incompatible with other information. And we do have some information installed in our subconscious that is not compatible with what we are trying on here. Hence the period of conflict within, during the time we are taking in new information and eradicating the old. That's persecution for righteousness sake. We are effectively being harassed by ourselves, within ourselves, because of the conflict between the old and the new.

But that's a good thing because when we are going through this struggle, we know we're getting somewhere. We have engaged the enemy. The Truth brings up anything unlike itself. And that is a very favourable state to be in because that struggle is part of getting the new anchored into your consciousness. It is well worth the struggle and it's to be expected. You are in a relationship with God even if it seems to be stormy. Any attempt at a connection to truth is a relationship with God. And any relationship with God is referred to as the kingdom of heaven. To be in this process of reconnecting is a blessed state.

Blessed are ye,
when men shall revile you, and persecute you,
and shall say all manner of evil against you
falsely,
for my sake.
Rejoice, and be exceeding glad:
for great is your reward in heaven
for so persecuted they the prophets
which were before you.

Everything we have looked at so far is about our inner world, and that's not going to change. Everything always comes from within. But the test is how we deal with the *outer* world. And the feedback from that outer world shows us how secure our newly established inner world is.

What is it like out there in the normal activity of the everyday world? What's it like with the other players on our stage that may not be of a like mind? Can we remain calm and at peace and true to our ideals in a world that is quite opposite? The final accomplishment to which we aspire is to hold to our Truth under any and all circumstances. And to do so *for my sake,* which is the Truth, represented in the Christ.

That ability is a good thing. Better than good. As I read it, we have to find a new category for happiness to contain this blessing. **'Rejoice, and be exceeding glad'**. Not exceedingly glad, but exceeding glad, meaning beyond glad; exceeding glad because the results are huge in terms of getting reconnected to the source of your being. And as the kicker: **for so persecuted they the prophets which were before you**. Anybody who has ever graduated from this school has gone through this.

So I for one found this last blessing particularly intriguing not to mention challenging. And that was just the understanding of it. Putting it into practice is still an ongoing exercise. So because of the challenge, I went through in understanding this, let alone practicing it, I'm going to use it as a little demonstration of what happens when we think. You might remember that I am strongly in favour of thinking. So here is a little peek behind the scenes into my thinking process.

The part that slowed me down and demanded that I think straight and read carefully was: **'falsely, for my sake'**. It was so simple really, when I saw it. But I found that understanding this was a little like tripping over one line in assembly instructions that 'anybody' can do, and then finally getting it. When I noticed the comma after falsely, I started to get it. That's when it dawned on me. I am being told here that when somebody is giving me a hard time, deservedly or otherwise, the trick is to hold to Truth, to not be disturbed, and to consciously keep Love in my heart no matter what's going on around me. If I can do that, I've got it made - big time. I've arrived. This is the goal. But if I can't do that, and I find myself reacting to negativity directed towards me, then that negativity directed toward me is not false. My reaction reveals that simple fact. The negativity directed towards me has found common ground with something within me that still needs releasing. Those old friends are still hanging around. Falsely was the keyword in the puzzle for me. Only after all manner of negativity directed to me does not find anything within me with which to connect, and thereby cause a reaction on my part, can that negativity be said to be directed falsely.

So there is thinking at its best, or at least my thinking at its best. Pondering, contemplating, and generally staying focused with a desire to understand is a process. And the real benefit of that process is that it invites the participation of spirit. A genuine quandary is a request for help. Spirit always responds when asked. Breakthroughs in thinking come from spirit, but it is only us who can initiate the process.

I have been given to understand that these opening statements are normally referred to as the Beatitudes. I have no quarrel with that. The incorporation of these Truths into our consciousness will certainly produce an attitude - an attitude that would create heaven on earth. An attitude of being: Beatitudes. How can you improve on that? Okay, I'm good with that. Henceforth, I will refer to these opening statements as the Beatitudes.

Ye are the salt of the earth:
but if the salt have lost his savour,
wherewith shall it be salted?
It is thenceforth good for nothing,
but to be cast out, and to be trodden under foot of men.
Ye are the light of the world.
A city that is set on a hill cannot be hid.
Neither do men light a candle, and put it under a bushel,

but on a candlestick;
and it giveth light unto all that are in the house.
Let your light so shine before men,
that they may see your good works
and glorify your Father
which is in heaven.

Salt is a preservative among other things. We maintain the condition of our lives here on earth by the quality of our consciousness. The savour is the quality of our being. If that quality is compromised in any way, then we lose our way and more. We lose our purpose, our meaning, and the awareness of our very identity. We lose our value. ***It is thenceforth good for nothing, but to be cast out, and to be trodden under foot of men.*** I'm glad those are not my words. A little strong, but maybe it's past time to mince words. It's time to wake up and get with it. As of this writing, the earth is in pain and the world's not doing so good. I can only hope that most people are a little more aware than I was with my absentminded activities that got the attention of a coyote.

It would seem that my common sense had to fall below the simple wisdom of a wild animal before I was shocked into putting my brain in gear and I started exercising my God-given ability to think. I don't think salting the earth the way I was doing it is what is meant here. No, we as the salt of the earth, means us as conscious beings and not daydreaming all the time. The quality of our lives and the conditions in our world are a reflection of the quality of our consciousness, individually and collectively.

The attitudes for being revealed in the Beatitudes is an outline of how to restore that quality of being, a method of removing all that obscures the Light. An open mind, willing to acknowledge all that obscures; the ability to connect to Source; looking within with determination; forgiveness with the goal of purification, culminating with the establishment of a peace that will withstand all opposition is the roadway suggested to get back to the true quality of our being.

Being the light of the world means being connected to our real selves and holding to that connection. We are the light of the world and when our attention is focused on Divine Truth, the light within us shines through automatically. Our real Selves are so bright and powerful, that once revealed, are impossible to hide. The Light of our beings, once rediscovered, is something we hold to easily and naturally. And it influences anyone and everyone, without us even trying or doing anything and without saying a word.

'Your good works' is the activity of working on your consciousness and removing all that obscures so that the Light may shine through for all to see. The keyword here is let. To let our light shine suggests that we have been inhibiting the light. The light is already there. Our job is to let the light shine through us by removing whatever has been blocking the light. We thereby glorify God, which reveals our purpose, our reason for being, and our true identity as children of God.

Do we see ourselves as we truly are as things stand now? No, not even close, or we wouldn't need to do this. I have a story that illustrates that very well. It's another story from elementary school.

This is a story about a great king. He was a benevolent ruler and very rich. One day a magical being came along and created a beautiful castle for the king. The castle was truly amazing and adorned with unbelievable riches. Every window border was lavished with rubies and diamonds, the likes of which were beyond the king's imagination. The whole thing was opulence personified. But the magical being left something out so that the king could contribute to this magnificent palace. One quarter of one of the many windows was left without the beautiful and priceless gems. This was left for the king to do, to complete the castle.

So of course the king gladly set about getting that done. He was so delighted at what he had been given that he was only too pleased to do his part, so he did not question the request. But even with all the king's vast riches, he could not manage to finish that window.

I don't think there were any consequences other than the appearance. I'm sure the king got to keep the palace anyway. That wasn't the point. The point was to get things in perspective so that the king could understand that, as rich and powerful as he was, it was minuscule compared to what he could be.

That story is a metaphor. We have at least that same discrepancy between what we are presently expressing and our potential. What we are accomplishing now is nothing compared to our potential - compared to what we can do when we are connected to our real power.

We are the custodians of the earth and the light of the world. It is through us that infinite potential is directed for the earth and our conditions. Supply is not the problem. Our problem is in knowing ourselves for what we really are. We have the authority to direct the mighty power of the universe wherever we choose. And yes, we did forget that somewhere along the way but that's why we have this reminder.

THE JOY OF SCHIZOPHRENIA

*Our Father
which art in heaven,
Hallowed be thy name.
Thy kingdom come.
Thy will be done on earth,
as it is in heaven.
Give us this day our daily bread.
And forgive us our debts, as we forgive our debtors.
And lead us not into temptation, but deliver us from evil;
For thine is the kingdom, and the power, and the glory,
forever.
Amen.*

I was very successful at a crisis and counseling centre where I spent a few years. As I progressed, I was given new and more interesting responsibilities, culminating in a position for which I was required to take two psychology courses at our local college.

I had not completed high school, but my adult status afforded me the luxury of enrollment without that prerequisite. And that was all fine, except that I was more than twice the age of the other students and a fair bit older than the professor. I don't think any of that would have mattered very much unless you sprinkle in a very different view of the world - a view that seriously questions the wisdom of conventional wisdom.

I found myself in a most interesting but profoundly disturbing framework. There I was, listening to a young mind steeped in the ways of the world, expounding those ways to even younger minds. The professor seemed to be quite confident in explaining the workings of our minds. And the minds that were exposed to this seemed to be absorbing it all without question. All except one.

I not only could not find anything within myself with which to match this incoming information, but rather I had a bigger problem to deal with. I was so astounded at the process of how the ways of the world are perpetuated, that I had very little attention left over to even try to understand how the others were able to make use of what was being said. I read the text at home because I needed the information to fulfill my purpose, but I really can't say that I actually took anything in, at least in terms of that which was intended in the content of the lectures.

Except once. One day our esteemed professor started the class by announcing that the answers to the previous day's quiz would now be given. And she asked if there was anyone who had not received one. Quiz? What quiz? I had not heard anything about any quiz. How could this be? I had never missed a class. So I asked a student near me and was informed that the quiz had been handed out in Tuesday's class. Tuesday's class? There's a class on Tuesday? Apparently. And apparently, as I came to find out later, there was a slight misprint on my schedule and I had been missing every other class right from the beginning. Of course, I had no way of knowing this. Having never made sense of the actual content of the lectures, how could I notice any gaps in continuity?

I was promptly given a quiz when I let it be known that I had not received one. At that point, it was late to be looking at it, but I glanced at it while the professor attended to another matter. There were 20 questions to be marked true or false. I looked at the first one and saw that it was dead easy. And so were the rest. So I quickly attended to this matter and got half of them done before the answers were to be given. I felt pretty good about it because I was confident that I would get 50%, given the fact that I got half of them done in that short time.

The answer was given to the first question: False. What? I got that wrong. How could that be? It was the easiest of them all. But before I could recover, the next answer was given and I got that wrong too. Near the end, I finally got one right. So that left me with one correct answer out of 20. A little off from that guaranteed 50% I had in mind. So I sat there in shock while the remaining answers were given.

My distressed state of mind didn't stop there. Oh no, our kindly professor would have us go public with our results. All who had a score between 15 and 20 were asked to raise their hands and further results were displayed in increments of 5 down to zero.

A surprisingly large number of hands were raised for the first category, the larger majority for the second category, and then the numbers dwindled quickly to the very last, in which only one lonely hand was displayed.

And our dear professor took note of this, would you believe? But not before we were given an explanation that finally made sense of this for me. The students who noticed my dunce hat looked at me in a very odd way but I didn't care because I suddenly realized that I had been vindicated by what the professor had just said.

We were told that the markings were somewhat arbitrary because the real purpose of the test was to see to what degree each of us takes our cues for our everyday decisions from the outer world, or from within ourselves. Are you an inner or outer person was what was being determined by the quiz.

Well, there is one thing I can promise you: A schizophrenic is an inner person!

But I found it very interesting that, even though we were told that the criteria for marking the questions were arbitrary, the scores were not changed. I, for example, should have been honoured as the top of the class. To her credit though, I will say that our dear professor smiled indulgently at me and used me as an example in other classes. That was something. But I think the main point was missed here. I think I should have been revered and that there should have been a statue of me placed at the main entrance of the college. Or at the very least, a plaque with my name on it. But none of these things happened. As far as I could see my contribution to reality caused barely a ripple.

On top of this, if I had had the time to look closely at the one question I got right, I would have got that one wrong too. If I had received the test at the previous lecture as I was supposed to, and had the time to look at it at my leisure, my score would have been zero.

Anyway, it wasn't long after that, that the discrepancy between the ways of the world and my ways became too evident and my career at the crisis centre came to an abrupt end. So I was relieved of my little stint in higher education.

But I did take two very important things with me that I've kept to this day:

The first was enormous respect for people with a formal education. I only got a little glimpse of it, but it was enough for me to see that there is a colossal amount of work entailed. I only had two courses going and I was swamped. Of course, I had my other duties at the centre to attend to as well, but still, it was nothing compared to what others with a full curriculum were taking on. I can only surmise that it takes a certain kind of dedication that I am unaware of to go through it all and get a degree. Mind you, I suppose it would be some contribution to motivation if you could actually believe in what you were taking in. But that was not something I could relate to.

The second thing I got to keep was my new status. I had always felt a little inadequate with the label of a high school dropout, but then all that changed. My little sojourn elevated my status. I may now refer to myself as a college dropout.

EPILOGUE

*And it came to pass,
when Jesus had ended these sayings,
the people were astonished at his doctrine:
For he taught them as one having authority,
and not as the scribes.*

Before starting to build a new fence with my father, we had to cut down some trees. We worked together, measuring, cutting, and loading the posts onto the wagon. We used a measuring stick to establish the lengths of the posts. It occurred to me that it would save a step if we used the post we had just cut as the measure for the next post since I was loading each post as we cut them and it would save me carrying that measuring stick around all the time. But my father explained if we did that, the slight mistake we might make could eventually compound and we might end up with a post that was two feet shorter than it should be, that the use of a constant for a measure was essential.

It was a very elementary lesson, so simple it's hardly worth mentioning, but it does represent the simple mistake we have made with this business of living our lives. It took a long, long time to get to where we are, to become so accustomed to hell that we accept it as more or less normal. It was indeed a very gradual process or we would have noticed it and done something about it long before this.

To do something that was not quite within the boundaries of Love, but so slight that it was not noticeable, as a measure for future behaviour, did not have much of an effect by itself, but over the centuries, it can and did have a devastating effect. Becoming accustomed to the nature of our world as it is at present, could only have come about in very tiny increments. But to anyone from the outside looking in, what we are doing now is ludicrous, and the unnecessary hardship must be beyond imagination.

To use the fence post analogy, we did not notice the gradual shortening of the posts even when they became shorter than the width of the wagon, which should have been obvious. And then when we constructed the fence without noticing that it was so low that the cows could jump over it, we still didn't get it. We blame the cows for being ornery rather than considering the possibility that we may have made an error somewhere along the line.

I am a little timid sometimes, but I have been trying to overcome that trait. Or at least put it aside while involved in this endeavour. So I hope it does not seem like I have been reticent about revealing what the constant of the universe is. And that that constant is what we really are. I have at least implied that if we must measure ourselves, what measure could there be but the one great constant in the universe? But of course, we don't need to measure ourselves at all. All we really need to do is accept ourselves for what we are. Against what background do you measure that which is perfect and Divine?

But we have, and we do measure ourselves all the time. And worse, the standard that we have become accustomed to has become so low that when we hear the real measure, we don't know what to do with it anymore. In fact, we have managed to distort and water down this simple truth over the centuries so much that it has lost most of its meaning. But that doesn't mean we can't find our way back. Nor does it mean that God has given up on us. As pointed out previously, there has always been a fail-safe in place to get us back on track. If all else failed, we would eventually come to a time when the Presence of God would become so strong that we couldn't miss it. Or go crazy. Which, as I have mentioned, accounts for all the rather bizarre goings-on in the world at the time of this writing.

The time of God's greater influence is now. But that greater influence does not take away our free choice. We still do, and will always, have the capability to turn our backs on God, which is turning our backs on ourselves. Turning our backs on God now, now that we have this far greater influence, is still possible, but of course, it has far greater consequences. This stronger influence of God only means that we have a lot more power at our disposal. It does not change our autonomy. It just makes the use of our power a lot more obvious, that's all. The benevolent influence of the universe is all around us now. And to ignore God, Love, the Truth of our being now, gives us the ability to raise havoc like never before. One who tends to be self-destructive will be successful. But Love will have its way, with or without anyone who's not willing to go along for the ride.

We have been delegated by God to manage our little corner of the world, wherever that might be. That delegation is given in full trust that we will use that power and authority consistent with the quality of that from which it was delegated. There is only one quality with which we are entrusted to work: The same quality by which all of creation was put in place. Therefore, the understanding and deployment of the Love that is within us, is the acceptance of that authority.

But if we misuse our authority by emanating anything but Love, our delegated authority must be rescinded. It is an automatic process put in place to protect the Divine harmony of the universe. We are allowed to make our mistakes as we learn and we can take as long as we want, but we can stop this silly bit about suffering with just a little more attention to what we are doing, anytime we want. As indicated, that long process of redefining ourselves in our own image has taken us so far away from reality that there is not much left resembling our true selves. And that's why we often don't understand the process of how, or why, or by what means, our delegated authority is rescinded - that process which usually takes a lifetime of misuse to complete and which is more commonly referred to as death.

This is not as bad as it sounds. Death has a bad name only because it is so misunderstood. I'm sure we'll see it a lot differently once we actually get there. And a little more understanding right now would give us respect for death and help us to appreciate the power of Love, Truth, the wonder of God, and the awesome magnificence of the universe.

Death is not punishment, or in any way meant to be a bad thing. Thank God for death, or we would stay in our mess forever. As I have mentioned before, death is just time out, that's all. We play hardball here and some of us need a little break once in a while. If we are unable to connect to Love or to learn how to deploy Love, a time-out has been provided so that we can get back to remembering the rules of the game. We only misunderstand death because we have learned to misunderstand Love, which means that we misunderstand everything of course. But we've already covered that.

Actually, the best approach to death is to get a little practice in ahead of time. That's what I did for retirement and it worked very well. I watched other people retire and I noticed that it was often fatal. So it was obvious to me that this was too much of a shock to the system all at once, especially late in life. So I practiced being retired for years to get the hang of it. I worked part-time for a while and I tried long periods of not working at all. And by the time it came to actual retirement, it was such a smooth transition that I hardly noticed it. So I've decided on the same approach to death. And so far it's working very well. It may be difficult for me to report on the final transition, but I'm getting so good at it that I think I can speculate on the last little bit and divulge it now.

Some people are very happy in retirement. So I don't see why retirement or death should be fatal with the proper approach. It just takes the right kind of practice that's all.

And if you've been paying attention, that practice is what we have been advocating here from beginning to end. The death of our old ways is the necessary prerequisite for allowing the entry of our true selves. So where are you going to get better practice than that? And to top it all off we're not giving up much. Giving up the ways of the world is probably easier than giving up smoking or drinking or any other addictions we have adopted as the surrogate to our addiction to hell. And even if that's a problem, there is an easy way to give up bad habits.

Probably the best advice I ever received from one of the great ones, was how to give up a bad habit. It was so simple it was laughable: Start the opposite good habit and as the new habit grows, the old habit will simply atrophy. But if that's challenging for some of our mundane habits, it will surely be easy for the ones we are advocating here. As the habit of Love grows, everything else has so little value that all our old ways just fall by the wayside as if they never were. And once we have died to our old ways, nothing else matters. Even the death of our bodies is trivial compared to the benefits of living in Love.

***

I did a little single parenting for a time. I had the great good fortune of regaining the privilege of caring for my son after a five-year absence. He was a little rebellious and for a good reason. He was very determined to go against the system, and me, and whatever he came across. It made perfect sense to me. How else could a child react when the basic requirements of life were either not provided or at best, the situation was such that these basic requirements were in question. He had developed a strong pattern that was destined for tragedy. All this was subconscious of course. He was convinced I would let him down again, and so he quite naturally did everything in his power to prove himself right. The determination of a child can be quite daunting.

But there were a few things that he did not know. For starters, he did not know that I understood all this and that I was fully aware that I had a challenge on my hands. But more importantly, what he could not possibly know is that I too was determined. I had a new kind of unwavering determination that can only come from at least some connection to Source. I considered his return to be a reprieve - a chance to undo the results of being derelict in my duties as a parent; the nightmare of watching his life go amuck, to which I had condemned myself. And he couldn't possibly know about the resulting anguish and soul searching that had been a large contribution to a change within myself. A change that had me entertaining other ways of defining life. And he couldn't know about the critical time of aloneness and severe illness that had led me to a fundamentally different approach with that difficult co-worker and how that little success had affected me. He could not know that I had a powerful determination based on my emerging trust in the great power of Love to heal all things.

So my son was up against a formidable opponent with his determination to fail and I was up for my greatest challenge and the greatest opportunity of my life. Without some understanding of the real truth of life, there would have been no contest. I don't even want to think about what could have been.

I understood that most of my work would be silent. Simple really. Return Love for all forms of rebellion, negativity, and or, any unloving behaviour. Love always wins. It's just a matter of time. But I did have my moments when my faith was severely tried. My big advantage of course was the natural Love of a parent for a child, even if that seemed to have been somehow lost in the shuffle between his mother and me for a time after I had tried her patience beyond human endurance. Still, there really is nothing like a second chance and the power of Love, when

Love is truly understood. I had had my success with what I called total acceptance and I held to that fiercely.

But then came a real test. One day, my son was particularly disobedient to the simple requirements that would keep us functional. We were walking home and he decided to go elsewhere. I commanded him to come with me but he disobeyed. We were in a situation and a location where I could not leave him alone and it seemed like force was the only option left to me. But something came over me and I flatly refused to play that game. I simp ly turned my back and silently walked away from him and did not look back.

I walked away physically but not mentally, not emotionally, and certainly not in my heart. While walking away I was with him with all the intensity of all the Love of my being. And after a while, he turned around and followed me without a word.

There was a silence between us the rest of the way home. I could see that he was quite mystified and finally he asked me with a very puzzled expression, "What would you have done if I had not come Dad?" I gave him an honest answer. I said, "I don't know". What I did not tell him is that my focus on Love was so strong that it did not leave room for consideration of anything else.

But let me intrude on my story here to quickly point out that I do not recommend this procedure. This was something that I was inspired to do in the moment and it worked. I could only have been inspired by Love because Love knew the results ahead of time. But this is not a formula to follow by any means. We must all do what we feel in the moment when we are in a crisis situation. Under no circumstances am I suggesting a particular solution to individual problems. This is only an example of the irresistible and magnetic power of Love when it is for real.

But to get back to this parenting thing: There came a day when I knew that it was all over. I always got a Father's

Day card every year. I guess that's kind of obligatory. But one year I got a very special surprise. I got a Mother's day card! That's when I knew that Love had claimed its victory.

And oh yes. I still get those Mother's day cards. When Love does its work, it's permanent.

***

Many years ago I watched an old movie starring Jerry Lewis. In one part of the show, he was playing the role of a would-be actor trying out for a part in a movie. He was given a classic line for his tryout: 'You say you love me, but you don't even know I'm alive.' And of course, ever the comedian, he repeated that line every way but right. He put the emphasis on different parts of the sentence every time so that it would give the line every meaning except what was intended. The part I remember the most was the last two words. I never knew you could say 'I'm alive' in so many different ways. The funniest one was when he made it sound like a question: 'I'm alive?! This line has become part of our family culture. We use it with good humour to this day.

But what about the actual intended meaning of that line? 'You say you love me, but you don't even know I'm alive.' It questions the sincerity of a declaration of Love. That's not a bad idea.

I've experienced a lot of misunderstanding around the meaning of Love and I've made some colossal errors in that area, quite a few small ones, and many mediocre ones. It must be impossible to wear God's patience out. Or could it be that He overlooks all the mistakes and only cares about the successes, no matter how small? By all reckoning, I should have been dead more than once with all my shenanigans, but I'm not.

I'm alive! You're alive! We're all alive and life is a Divine privilege! Especially now that we have such enormous opportunities on planet earth. We are being reminded of what we have forgotten about ourselves.

Maybe what is so difficult for us to understand is that Love requires nothing. There is no price for God's Love. Love only wants to Love. The opportunity to Love is Love's reward. This means that our challenge in the stage we are at is to develop the ability to receive. We need to raise our expectations to something way beyond our present state. And when we start to really understand, we will need a new category for happiness which was so clearly pointed out in the last Beatitude: ***Exceeding glad.*** Beyond this and that and the glad and sad of normal living, we are to live in Joy.

THE FINAL THEREFORE

> **Therefore
> whosoever heareth these sayings of mine,
> and doeth them,
> I will liken him unto a wise man,
> which built his home upon a rock:
> And the rain descended, and the floods came,
> and the winds blew,
> and beat upon that house;
> and it fell not:
> for it was founded upon a rock.
> And everyone that heareth these sayings of mine,
> and doeth them not,
> shall be likened unto a foolish man,
> which built his house upon the sand:
> And the rain descended, and the floods come,
> and the winds blew,
> and beat upon that house;
> and it fell: and great was the fall of it.**

Construction is going on just outside my window. The street is being torn up and rebuilt, it's noisy, and it's a little aggravating. I used to work in road construction and I'm glad I kept my ear protection apparatus from those days. Rather interesting work actually, and aside from the noise, it's messy and can even be confusing at times. It takes a lot of planning and special kinds of people to get the job done. I was involved with moving the equipment around, so I saw it all. It sure wasn't routine - way too many variables for that and always something unexpected coming up. I was very impressed with the people who made it all happen. Sometimes it looked like the job would never get done, but the day would eventually come when it was complete and beautiful to behold.

That noisy construction caused me to use my ear protection while writing. I thought that the noise was a bit much and some of it even unnecessary. The normal sounds of construction are not that bad. Most of the machines have good mufflers and even the sound of material being moved is tolerable. But it's those annoying beepers that are meant to warn you when a machine is backing up, that go too far. They are meant to compete with the noise of the engine to get your attention and they do that very well. But when there is a constant to and fro, and when several machines are working at once, those infernal beepers seem mostly to be competing with each other. Certainly, this constant beeping has long since been ignored by the workers. But if they are not annoying to the construction workers they are certainly annoying to me. Surely that's taking a supposedly good thing to the point where it loses its meaning.

Let's see if I've got this right. The workers wear ear protection because of the excess noise of construction. And the beepers have to be loud enough to be heard through ear protection. Did I miss something? The sound of construction would be tolerable without that additional sound proclaiming to the world that construction is taking place. Everybody on the street knows about it. Do you have to announce it to the world continually, to the point of obnoxious irritation!?

Still, the benevolence of the universe sees to it that nothing is ever wasted. I probably would not have worn my ear protection had it not been for those 'bleep, bleep' beepers. But after using my ear protection to reduce the effects of that noise, it occurred to me to use that same protection during the times when I try to shut my mind off. And it worked. It worked much better than I expected. I was able to shut my mind off like never before. If it wasn't for those beepers that I have been raging about, I might never have stumbled onto the great benefit of taking ear protection to a new level. I have been given a great gift towards achieving my highest goal from an unexpected source. I was not very pleased at the distraction of that construction when it first started, but now I can't help seeing it just a little differently. Such a simple thing, ear protection. Why didn't I think of that before? Sound is the one above all of our senses that keeps us connected to the outside world, and here I have been given a simple method of helping me to shut the world off. I've had this ear protection thing around for years but it never occurred to me to use it to enhance meditation. All adversity yields something good because there is only good.

And now sitting here watching their procedures while wearing ear protection, I realize there is a clear parallel between construction and the rebuilding of the constitution of our individual kingdoms and of the collective change going on in the world. The mind gets noisy when you stir it up with new information and that's happening on a larger scale in the world. Many people are making a lot of noise trying to keep things the same even if they don't realize it.

I thought the street was fine but maybe the people who keep the city functional know something I do not. And maybe there is something about ourselves that we do not know about either. There is a higher knowing that would suggest that we could become aware of how inadequate our world is and that there is some rebuilding that needs to be done. Actually, the information I have is that the reconstruction of the situation in the world is a little overdue. But it is underway, even if we haven't all noticed it yet. And it is noisy, messy, and definitely a little confusing. And there are a lot of us making way more noise than necessary during the process. The whole world needs to know about our individual problems as much as it needs to know that my street is being rebuilt.

But the rebuilding of our world has to be done - noisy or otherwise. The highway we have been traveling on can't take us home no matter how much we patch it up. Not to mention the fact that it has a dead end. So ready or not, we are rebuilding our world. Even those who do not know about it are helping by subconsciously resisting it. That resistance draws greater attention to the need for change.

And as a by-product of change, we are taking fear to an extreme. Because we are accustomed to being motivated and working in terms of fear, part of the progression from hell to heaven is a transition period that accentuates fear. During this period we are translating the new emerging reality in terms of fear. Therefore, for now, we are making rules based on fear to protect ourselves from the very things that fear brings about. This is a necessary interim step to highlight fear that it may be exposed for what it truly is: The causative factor of all our problems. The absurdity of wearing ear protection and then deliberately making a sound loud enough to be heard over the ear protection is a symbol of our times. We are building a new world. And it is messy, noisy, confusing and there is a lot of misunderstanding. But the day will come when all the mess, noise, misunderstanding, and confusion will end and it will be obvious that all that construction was worthwhile. More than worthwhile; a lot more. So we need these absurdities for now. What we are doing is necessary. No matter what we do, we are all learning from it.

Each of us is responding or reacting to the increasing influence of spirit in our own way. We are doing something, even if it's wrong. What some people are doing is obviously wrong. But is it really wrong when we take what has always been implied to an extreme for all to see? Is it really wrong when corruption is exposed for all to see? We are making the change by doing, one way or the other. Doing what doesn't work is an essential part of change. No matter what we do, we learn by doing. We are all in this together. The ones who are confused and making all the noise are making just as big a contribution to change as anybody else; maybe more so. It is doing that creates the change in us.

Individually or collectively, doing what doesn't work is an essential part of learning. It's all part of getting back to what does work.

In fact, the one thing that can accelerate change is to remember that we learn by doing. True understanding can only come from doing. And after we are all through with doing what doesn't work, when we run out of things to do that don't work, there will be nothing left except what does work. And then we can repeat what works until it becomes who we are. That repetitive doing is more commonly referred to as practice. It takes practice. Even if it's clumsy at first, we do. We do until we have it where we want it. It has to go through the system to be installed and be a permanent part of us. Doing is what installs it on the hard drive. Without putting these things into practice, we have nothing at all. Then it's just information that is forgotten as soon as something else demands our attention. It evaporates in the moment. Information by itself is useless unless it is practiced until it becomes a state of being.

Life without the truth of our being installed within us takes away our sense of being; whereas, life based on the truth of being makes life understandable. Then being just is. Then, not being is no longer a possibility. We have dealt with and answered the question of being or not being once and for all. 'To be or not to be?' seems to be the eternal question but it is not. It is only a question as long as we are in this limited condition we have created. The very thing we are working our way out of. Once we have installed what we have here to the point of permanency and therefore wisdom, we are left with the singularity of being. Being the human beings we were meant to be without the question. We are at the point of figuring everything out. I hope Hamlet doesn't mind, but we can't put off answering that question much longer.

***

My modern computer automatically corrects my spelling as I go along. Except where my spelling is too far off, which happens quite frequently, and then it just underlines the word in red. The computer does all it can to clean up my mistakes, but I get a little careless sometimes. And when I get too far off, I have to go back and pay attention and see if I can get the spelling at least close enough so that spell check can fix it. There are three stages to this correction apparatus. In the first stage, spell check cleans up my mistakes as I go along. In the second stage, it underlines the word in red. At that point, I can highlight that word, click on spell-check and I may be offered several possibilities to click on. But in the third stage, when I'm too far away from the correct spelling, there is nothing that can be done to help me. It just comes up, 'not in dictionary, no suggestion'.

I usually wait until I have a page or two or even a whole document if I'm on a roll, and then check everything at once. That often brings interesting results. For one thing, there are usually a lot of words underlined, and too, I notice that I repeatedly misspell some of the same words. Of course, I could look at the correct spelling and learn something if I wanted to but I don't bother. But it isn't just spelling. My typing is not what it could be because I am forever getting ahead of myself. Not very efficient really. Bad habits are hard to break. So much easier to learn the right way in the beginning. Mind you, I have a good excuse, I didn't learn to type until I was in my seventh decade. But for some strange reason, my computer does not take that into account. It makes no allowance for seniority or age or anything else I can come up with. I get discounts and all kinds of special treatment as a senior, but my computer refuses to afford me that kind of respect. I may have to complain to Bill Gates.

But even with that limitation, my computer is very impressive for a man-made machine. Our modern technology is getting ever closer to perfection. It is the natural goal that we are aspiring to, knowingly or otherwise. But even if we do get to perfection with our technology, that technology will still have one big limiting factor. It will never be able to think. Nor does the great and always perfect intelligence of the universe have that ability. The Holy Spirit, even though it is perfect and all-knowing, cannot think. It only knows and it knows all because it is the mind of God. But it cannot think as we do.

When you communicate with a computer as in, let's say a bank statement, I have noticed the indifference in the communication that comes back to me; even if I have made an error or even if my financial situation is in a disastrous state. And that's the way the universe has to run. No matter what our situation is, even to the point of being on death's door, the laws must take place. There could not be any leeway in universal laws or we would have chaos. ***For verily I say unto you, Till heaven and earth pass, one jot or one title shall in no wise pass from the law, till all be fulfilled.*** God is certainly not indifferent to us but He had to set the laws of the universe up to be impartial or we couldn't have complete autonomy. How's that for Love?

I have not been trying to keep it a secret that we are the thinking part of the universe. And I may even have alluded to the fact that I am a strong advocate of thinking. That's all it takes to get creation going. Everything is in place. It's all set up so that we can't miss. Perfection is just waiting to be released into wherever we choose to set our attention. There is only positive. Creation is positive. That's why it's called creation. It's not called destruction. Creation can only come about through positive activity. Creation was all put together by Love. There is only Love. All else in evidence comes about through misunderstanding; by the use of perfect power to create imperfectly. And that little misunderstanding is what we have been trying to clear up.

We make a difference no matter what we do, with or without Love. What influence do we want to have? What we think and do influences everything. ***As a man thinketh***. But that's a two-way street. Even though the Holy Spirit cannot think as we think of thinking, it is an influence. The sun influences me and will even change the colour of my skin. It is a benevolent influence but it cannot decide on how long I will stay outside. It cannot decide whether or not I will get sunburned. There is a universal force and influence that is constantly providing our every need but it cannot make decisions. It's all set up and ready to go. All it needs is a conscious direction to be activated and released into use. And that mighty influence insists on perfection and ultimately will not have it any other way. It's called Love. We are the part of it that directs where and what that force will manifest. We are learning how it works so that we may take an active, direct, and conscious role in that activity. We make mistakes as we go along, but that all-knowing perfect force is ever at the ready to underline our mistakes that we may have another look and get it right.

Underlining everyday living are consequences. Whatever we think and do has a result; we qualify the great force of the universe in every moment. That's a given by the definition of being human, or more accurately, children of God. We have the keys to the kingdom to use as we see fit. Our thoughts are hooked into the universal mind for better or for worse. All we have to do is connect the dots and learn so that we can stop this silly business of suffering and get on with co-creating with God as we are meant to. In perfection. And in tune with Divine Harmony at all times by being connected to our true nature, understanding completely without the possibility of misunderstanding. There is a point after enough practice where the influence of spirit is so strong that it is impossible to make a mistake. Jesus was and is the personification of that. And He said in the plainest words possible: *'What I do, ye shall do, and greater things*

shall ye do.' He knew without a shadow of a doubt, that this is our destiny. And he knew that the day would come when it would be ever so much easier to understand and to learn and become all we are meant to be. He knew when that time would be and that's one of the reasons why He came at a time far enough back so we would have plenty of time to make our mistakes and get ready for the final push. He even told us in the beginning that this is the final update. This is as good as it gets in terms of being given what we need to get our act together.

The influence of spirit is so strong now that everything around us reminds us of a better way. And it certainly is evident in our technology. Even my generation is noticing it, though we may struggle with it.

My older sister, for example, has a love/hate relationship with her computer. It took a lot of insistence on the part of a younger sibling to get her to even consider using such a contraption. And then it took a massive amount of coaching on the part of this same sibling. Not to mention a fair bit of insistence to overcome resistance. But even with that somewhat ambiguous attitude, our senior student of technology did get on track with a certain ability to take command of this scary machine.

I think the reason some of us older people have trouble with technology is that the type of work involved does not have the immediacy we are accustomed to. There was a particular comment that my sister made that sums up the frustration of those of us who did not grow up with computers. She wished she could just get in there and grab something and make the necessary adjustments. That's it right there!

We are used to tangible things, things that we can get our hands on and make the changes we want. But that's not how computers work. A computer is a machine that responds to commands, but the activity involved is within a closed system that is effectively hidden from us. We do have hands-on, but it's a very different concept of hands-on. We no longer have that direct contact with the actual activity that accomplishes a given end. Working with a computer is not like writing by hand or filing documents in a folder and then physically putting them in a cabinet. That we understand. If we lose a document, we just hunt until we find it. But now, with a computer if you lose something or if something goes wrong, it's a whole new ball game. You have to stop and figure it all out and check and see what errors you made, which can be a painstaking and very frustrating experience. Not to mention mentally taxing to the point of confusion. It can be all very trying and can easily lead one to give up and call a grandchild to come and fix the problem. But that latter solution still keeps us at arm's length from being computer literate and keeps us away from the understanding of how the world functions these days.

Machines did our work and we could see the process in most cases. A machine that moved hay on the farm did the same as we could do by hand. It just did it a lot better and was more efficient. Operating the machine entailed manipulating controls and watching the results. But computers have placed us in a completely different relationship with work. So much so, that we almost have to redefine work. By commanding our computers to do our bidding, we are doing just that, making commands. Commands activate a series of events to give us the desired result. Granted the method of accomplishing this was coming for a while, but that last step to the computer age has been huge.

It's all great, but it's considerably more demanding in terms of mental accuracy. And that's the part that's so frustrating to those of us who are not as computer literate as we might be. The feedback we get when we make an error can be a little humbling. It forces us to re-examine the commands we have given when we do not get the results we expect. Or blame the computer; but most of the time that just won't wash. Most of the time, when we backtrack through the whole process, we find one tiny error that we have made in our commands and probably conflicting commands that cancel each other out. Computers demand a kind of accuracy in thinking never before required. And that's what is so annoying and that's what we oldies don't want to admit. There is a new level of mental competence required in these times that we just never knew about in other times. The computer age has completely changed how we function and it's making us a lot more honest.

I have wasted so much time getting nowhere with my computer that I have had to institute a strict policy with my endeavours: If at first I don't succeed, the hell with it. So let's just forget about the older generation. We don't represent the future anyway. The concerns of those of us who have difficulty adjusting are only useful to demonstrate the magnitude of the change going on in the world. It is quite inspiring to see how we, as a whole, have adapted so quickly to a completely new way and a higher level of thinking.

Children, of course, are into computer games now. This seems to be the way that children are introduced to our technological world. Just like we used to play with toy trucks or whatever, and would eventually take on the corresponding occupations. I think all those games and the like are called virtual reality. I was shocked when I first heard that term. I misunderstood at first. It seemed to me that we were giving our children something to do that replaced reality. And I still think that to some extent. There is some of that in it and it does worry me, but children are just emulating adults like they always have and they are learning the essentials through their play like they always have.

Young people take to the computer age like a duck to water. They work with computers as if there never was any other way to function. As always, the younger generation comes in with an underlying understanding of the new emerging reality. They of course do not know this on a conscious level, but they don't need to. The influence is strong and they are strong and they trust what they feel and it all works for them. Some are consciously aware of it and some are not, but it doesn't matter. All are aware to some extent and all are participating in the process of building a wonderful new reality on planet Earth. Computer experts are very motivated and delighted by their ability to understand. And that's as it should be. They are doing a great job. It's very gratifying to be an expert in the field that represents the future. And more power to you. I for one can't do without you.

But there is a little more than a generation gap involved here. We are taking everything to a higher level - much higher, the highest. We are going to take this know-how to a new kind of knowing that will make our technology look elementary. Our new understanding is taking us in a direction other than that which is obvious. There is a greater purpose being played out. What computers are really doing for all of us, aside from making our lives a lot easier, is preparing us for a future so vastly different than our recent past, that even young people will be awed by it. Even the brightest and most computer literate of the new generation could be in for something far beyond their expectations.

The greater reality unfolding is that we have translated the increasing influence of spirit to a replication of spirit through our technology. This is all part of spirit seeping in and influencing us very quietly without notice. We are preparing ourselves for an understanding of the workings of spirit. It is truly a wondrous thing that is going on and it is truly a wondrous world emerging. What we are really doing with our technology is taking our knowing to a new level of understanding, *about ourselves.*

There is a similarity between the workings of spirit and the mechanism of a computer and that similarity is just enough to give us a little preview and the very necessary practice. We are indeed once removed from the workings of spirit, just as we are once removed from the workings of a computer. And it can cause the same kind of frustration that my sister expressed with her desire to 'get in there and grab the thing'. But getting in there and grabbing is not how spirit works. You can't grab spirit with your hands. The commands we give have an effect even when we are not aware of the mistakes we have made in our commands. We are learning a very important thing by the mental accuracy demanded of us in working with our modern technology. We are learning to be more mentally astute, to be more consciously aware, and to be alert to the possibility that we may be making conflicting or inaccurate demands. Working with a computer demands a kind of honesty that is serving us very well in learning to work with spirit.

That's the real benefit of our computer age. We are learning to be very clear in our thinking. But more importantly, we are gaining the ability to concentrate. I have noticed that when computer experts are engaged in the more demanding activities like programming, their attention is so fixed that you can't distract them even with a forceful intrusion. That kind of concentration is a most important prerequisite to connecting to spirit. If we can learn to concentrate well enough to shut out all the distractions of the world when we are trying to focus on spirit, we've got a good start. So the practice it takes to gain the necessary ability to concentrate when working with a computer is an enormous help.

And more, we are learning to trust; we are getting used to that once removed phenomenon. It is a wonderful practice to work with a computer and the exacting way it works. As mentioned, my generation often finds those exacting demands quite frustrating, but young or old, we all have this opportunity to get a little preview into an accurate view of cause and effect. We can get a glimpse of how spirit works by working with our ever-improving technology. We are learning that critical step of becoming aware that it is our commands that activate the real power.

We cannot be separate from spirit because we are spirit, but for all practical purposes, the barrier of being physical presents a barrier to spirit which keeps us once removed from the literal hands-on of cause and effect. So it's just a matter of time before we see the obvious. That we, defined as physical beings, do nothing. I didn't make that up: **'I do nothing; The Father within me, He doeth the work.'**

This could be the biggest step to understanding and reconciling to spirit and that's why I mentioned that even the young people could be in for a surprise. We are taking that critical step towards trusting that our commands will have the effect we desire. And coming to that realization that it is often not the fault of the computer when something goes wrong, can take us to the realization that it is never the fault of spirit when we do not get the results we expect.

A computer may malfunction but not so with spirit. There can be times when we can blame our computers for a faulty outcome but we do not have that luxury with spirit. Spirit responds with 100 % accuracy every time. There is nobody and no thing to blame. Of course, the good thing about that is that you know where to look to solve the problem. Just like now when I have a problem with my computer it's probably something I did, I know that when I have a problem with ultimate cause and effect, it's *always* something to do with my commands or the absence thereof.

So if we keep going the way we are, are we going to stumble onto the ultimate technology? I'm told that the scientific world has, or is close to, isolating the smallest particle. But apparently there is a problem because this particle seems to be allusive. It would seem that the simple act of observation has an effect on this particle. Hmm. Now what's that all about? And where is that taking us? If observation changes matter then we really are onto a revolutionary change in how we believe everything works.

And the last I heard, a name for this particle had not been decided on, although it has been jokingly referred to as the God particle. Well if it really is affected by the simple act of observation maybe that joking reference is not as far off as it would seem. That's pretty basic to all the information we have here. 'As a man thinketh' comes to mind. Is that the big connection? And what does that say about cause and effect? Maybe science and religion aren't as far apart as we have been led to believe. Where are we going with our ever-improving technology? Are we indeed getting to the ultimate technology? Are we starting to notice God's technology? And if so, can we really compare our man-made technology to how nature works? Well yes. What other model do we have to work from, even if we don't acknowledge the source of our inspiration?

So if we accept that infamous particle as the God particle and then go on to reason that since all other particles are made of that, what particle is not of God? And if we want to keep going with that reasoning, what we call our world, or our planet is also a God particle. Just a little bigger that's all. So if that smallest particle is influenced by us and since it makes up everything, what then is not influenced by us? It seems to me that as God beings, how we could not influence a God particle would be a better question.

In the meantime, we are making good use of our technology. Even to the point of having what seems like two-way verbal exchange. I am amused by the way some of us communicate with our computers. Or at least it seems like communication (I am aware that there is software available whereby one may give verbal commands to a computer, but that's not what I am referring to here). I am referring to how some of us actually talk to our computers a lot like we might talk to our car when it isn't running right. I don't think it's too uncommon to hear someone make derogatory remarks directed at a computer when the results of one's efforts do not meet the expected outcome.

Is this the way we communicate with God? Well yes, it often is, even if we do not think of it as that. In either case, with the computer and with God, I do not think the quality of the communication to which I have referred yields any positive results. Both computers and God are rather exacting in their demands that we do things correctly - one considerably more than the other. And neither has the software to translate our feelings of frustration into anything constructive.

When we give commands and something goes wrong with some automated system that we use in our everyday interaction with others, it is usually referred to as a system error. And that's fine, but it has to involve human error somewhere along the line. Even if it's within the technology itself, if we look long enough, we are going to find a human error. But there is no system error in God's technology. That's why we call it natural as in nature. It is God's nature to work perfectly. Any imperfection we experience in our lives is not a systems error. Any imperfection we experience is an error in the commands we make to the perfect system within nature.

We can't expect our technology to be anything like the perfect creation by God, but we could notice that we are being divinely inspired, that our technology is coming ever closer to the way everything in nature works. The function of computers can give us a bit of an idea of how we function and could even give us a bit of a clue to that seemingly missing link to understanding our autonomy.

As we install the information we have been working on here into our minds, we can compare it to the process of installing new information into a computer. When we set up something new into our computers, something in addition to or instead of what we already have, there is usually a message on the screen that is something like this: 'Do you wish to keep this or default to the old program'? Default is the keyword. Until the new information we have exposed ourselves to on the conscious level is established, firmly established into the subconscious, our minds will automatically default to what has been previously established. Deleting an old program from our subconscious minds is not as easy as a click with the mouse. The kind of change we are advocating here is a fundamental change in the definition of our identity. And that's where the comparison to a computer falls short. We can only go so far with our comparison, but just far enough to get some critical understanding. We do have an extremely sophisticated mechanism within us that serves us unfailingly and perfectly. But it will only respond to the supreme command of the universe rather than the click of the mouse before it will allow a change. We are Divine and it takes no less than Divine intervention to bring us back to that realization. We must use the power of our Divinity to restore our Divinity.

It takes a bit of work to completely revamp the kingdom and get it back on track and click into our Divinity, but nothing will be permanently in place until we do exercise that Divine ability and that Divine right. We have the right and the ability to use the one and only power that commands all things. We have the right and ability to Love. We have the right and ability to Love ourselves, which includes forgiveness. We have the right and the ability to direct Love where we will. And that ability to Love ourselves and all others and all there is, is synonymous with being connected to our power. Nobody can do this for us. Not even God. Our sacred autonomy is supreme because of our true identity and we can only reconcile to our true identity on our own because of our sacred autonomy. Know the truth and the truth will not let your mind default to the ways of the world.

This means that a love/hate relationship with a computer is a good place to start to get a little practice on deleting the hate part. I have noticed that feelings of anger or frustration with my computer don't help. Rather, I suspect that these negative feelings keep me separate from the inspiration that might otherwise give me some insight as to how to solve the problem.

***

We are indeed addressing the big questions these days. Big questions like Love or the absence thereof. We are delving into questions about the smallest particle, cause and effect, and what we are. We are starting to find out that there is a lot more to us than we thought.

Of course, I have never doubted that. I have always had dreams and imaginings that go right off the scale. I have very lofty aspirations. And that's to be expected with my condition. Delusions of grandeur go with the territory. But of course, these are not delusions to me, or I wouldn't have the condition. My ambitions go far beyond the simple task of putting my thoughts into the written form. Oh yes, these few words are pretty small potatoes compared to my real ambitions. My wildest dreams are indeed of greatness and they do indeed include grandeur. My definitive desires have to do with making a contribution and a change for the better to the mass consciousness. By freeing myself of my personal limitations, I will remove that from the mass consciousness and thereby make a *real* contribution. *Then my light will so shine that it cannot be hid.* That's greater than anything tangible like a book. Heal yourself and you heal the world. That is truly my ultimate dream and the only worthy goal from our present stance.

Only a normal person can refer to my dreams of grandeur as delusion, but that doesn't mean that a normal person can't aspire to grandeur. The grandeur of our beings becomes evident once we have all this information made available to us here, firmly installed into our consciousness to the point that we do all these things automatically.

That's why it's likened to building a house on a solid foundation. These teachings are the material. The incorporation of them into our consciousness is the building of the house. Then you have a frame of reference within which to experience being, based on that which is not changeable.

We have all felt separate from one another to some degree because we lost our common thread. Our seeming separation from God has influenced each of us differently and therefore made us all see the world in unique ways. But even though these ways have become distorted, we do have as many viewpoints as people. And we are indeed meant to express uniquely and differently, but with one very important similarity. We, with all our unique and different perspectives, are unique and different expressions of God. And so of course we do have a common thread. It's the common thread throughout creation without which creation couldn't exist. And each of us can get back to that which is common to us all, anytime and in any way we want.

The words we have been exposed to here are meant to awaken us to our knowing and to our truth. And as they become our own, we are building a new structure within which to experience our being. Your unique truth is based on the solid rock of the universal truth of Love to be expressed in your unique way

www.ingramcontent.com/pod-product-compliance
Lightning Source LLC
Chambersburg PA
CBHW051934290426
44110CB00015B/1968